Gelson Aguiar da Silva Moser
Zuila Mª F. Carvalho
Denise C. Moser Aguiar

Functional Independence for People with Paraplegia

Gelson Aguiar da Silva Moser
Zuila Mª F. Carvalho
Denise C. Moser Aguiar

# Functional Independence for People with Paraplegia

## Results and Associated Factors

ScienciaScripts

**Imprint**

Any brand names and product names mentioned in this book are subject to trademark, brand or patent protection and are trademarks or registered trademarks of their respective holders. The use of brand names, product names, common names, trade names, product descriptions etc. even without a particular marking in this work is in no way to be construed to mean that such names may be regarded as unrestricted in respect of trademark and brand protection legislation and could thus be used by anyone.

Cover image: www.ingimage.com

This book is a translation from the original published under ISBN 978-613-9-60685-6.

Publisher:
Sciencia Scripts
is a trademark of
Dodo Books Indian Ocean Ltd. and OmniScriptum S.R.L publishing group

120 High Road, East Finchley, London, N2 9ED, United Kingdom
Str. Armeneasca 28/1, office 1, Chisinau MD-2012, Republic of Moldova, Europe
Printed at: see last page
ISBN: 978-620-7-29610-1

# DEDICATORY

To **Evelise,** my wife, companion and great encourager on this journey.


To my children **Isabela** and **Breno**, for the time I didn't dedicate to them, but which I now realise was worth it!


To my parents, **João Francisco** and **Francisca,** and to my siblings (Marlei, Nilton, Ailton, Flávio, Caio and Sibéle), who, although far away, have always supported me throughout this journey.


My advisor, **Profª Drª, Zuíla Maria de Figueiredo Carvalho**, for her teachings, encouragement, friendship over these five years and for believing in my intellectual potential, thank you very much!

# ACKNOWLEDGEMENTS

Although I don't profess a formal religion, but I have always feared and had faith in God, I thank him for his constant presence in my life.

To the professors, staff and colleagues of the Postgraduate Programme, who contributed to my constant learning, and to the Federal University of Ceará, a public source of knowledge, especially "Ju", the person in charge of the reception desk at the Department of Nursing - UFC.

The Sarah Network of Rehabilitation Hospitals, especially Dr° . Aloysio Campos da Paz Júnior and Drª Lúcia Willadino Braga, directors of the institution, who allowed this study to be carried out there.

The Sarah-Fortaleza Rehabilitation Centre, especially Dr Thereza Christina de Lara Alvim, for recognising the importance of the research.

To the Scientific Committee of the Sarah-Fortaleza Rehabilitation Centre, composed of Dr° . Daniel de Paula Lima e Oliveira Lopes, Dr° . Ênio Alberto Comerlato and Dr° .Mauro Nakayama, for their valuable contributions and enrichment of the work.

To the Nursing Management of the Sarah-Fortaleza Rehabilitation Centre, made up of nurses Kátia Isabel Lima Lemos and Andréia Socorro Idalino Janebro, for their encouragement.

To my colleagues in the Spinal Cord Injury Programme, for their understanding, support and encouragement on this journey, especially my leader and friend Linda Arair C. de Alencar, who worked a real "miracle" in adjusting my work schedule.

To my friends Adolfo, Adilina, Fábio, Marta, Deyse, Juliana, Heloísa, the "Dedés" and Mrs Ivone, for their constant support and encouragement.

To my fellow nurses from the spinal cord injury programme, Cristiane, Antonio Lucieudo, Cristina Janaína, Guldemar, Mara Lúcia, Rosimeire, Tarciana, Uverlange, Valéria and Winner and nursing assistants Celma and Vânia Kelly for their support and cheering me on during this important stage in my life.

To the administrative assistant Daniken Fermon, for his IT assistance.

To my friends, Janaina Vall and Jean Felizardo, for their invaluable help in formatting the work, contributions and corrections.

To the statisticians Sandro Barbosa de Oliveira and Cruiff Emerson Pinto da Silva, for their invaluable help in analysing the data, criticisms and suggestions, especially to Cruiff for accompanying us at every stage of the work.

To the grammar, style and sentence construction proofreader, Profº . Dr Vianney Mesquita, from the Federal University of Ceará and the Ceará Academy of the Portuguese Language, for his sound advice and teacherly substitutions of words and expressions.

To the patients with spinal cord injuries, who make me realise every day what a small achievement means!

## THE TRUTH...

The door to the truth was open,

But he only let half a person through at a time.

So it wasn't possible to reach the whole truth,

Because half the people who came in

He only had the profile of a half-truth.

And its second half

He also returned with half a profile.

And the half profiles didn't match up.

They broke down the door. They broke down the door.

They reached the bright place

Where the truth was blazing.

It was divided into halves

Different from each other.

They even discussed which half was more beautiful.

Neither of them was totally beautiful.

And they had to choose. Everyone chose according to their whim, their illusion, their short-

sightedness.


Carlos Drummond de Andrade (*Corpo*, Record)

## EXERCISE

Science, love, wisdom.

Everything lies far away, always

- immensely out of our reach.

The atom falls apart,

You control the tears,

abysses can now be overcome

- But he immediately falls to his stomach with his eyes closed,

and it's a little secret

about a big secret.

We will be sad for a long time to come,

Although with a noble sadness,

The sun and the moon

every day they find

only silence reflected in the mirror,

in this long exercise of the soul.

Cecília Meireles, 1955.

**TEACHING**


My mum thought I was studying

the finest thing in the world.

It's not

The finest thing in the world is feeling.

That day in the evening, his father was cooking,

she spoke to me:

"Poor chap, he's been working hard until this hour."

He put bread and coffee away, left a pot on the hob with hot water.

He didn't talk to me about love.

That word of luxury.


Adélia Prado

## THE MIRACLES


The miracle is not giving life to an extinct body,

or light to the blind, or eloquence to the mute...

Or change pure water into red wine...

It's a miracle that they believe all this!

Mario Quintana


If you can look, look. If you can see, notice. (*Book of Advice*)

# SUMMARY

Spinal cord injury can lead to limitations for the individual, but a rehabilitation programme that assesses functional gain allows monitoring throughout the course of rehabilitation. The aim of this study was to evaluate the results obtained with the application of the Functional Independence Measure (FIM) in people with paraplegia undergoing a rehabilitation programme; associating these findings with the following variables: age, gender, time, level and etiology of the injury, classification of the injury according to the ASIA (*American Spinal Injury Association*) criteria, length of hospitalisation, education and complications (pressure ulcers, heterotopic ossification, spasticity and neuropathic pain). To this end, a quantitative cross-sectional, retrospective, descriptive study was carried out, analysing 228 medical records and the scores obtained using the MIF Scale. Analyses were carried out using specific tests using SPSS (*Statistical Package for the Social Science*) *software*, version 13 for *Windows*. The results showed that, among the variables studied, there is a direct relationship between age, time since injury, motor level, length of hospitalisation and hospitalisation with a companion and gain in independence (p< 0.05). There was also an inverse relationship between the classification of the injury (AIS A, B, C, D or E) and functional gain (p< 0.05). Functional assessment in people with spinal cord injuries, using the Functional Independence Measurement Scale, makes it possible to monitor functional gain in people undergoing a rehabilitation programme.

**Keywords:** rehabilitation, paraplegia, activities of daily living, nursing.

# SUMMARY

# CHAPTER 1

# INTRODUCTION

Diseases and injuries to the Central Nervous System (CNS) and their consequent sequelae are becoming more frequent and prevalent in contemporary society, due to the general ageing of the population, the increased survival of patients as a result of better care in the acute phase of diseases, and also due to the increase in violence and resulting traumatic injuries (GREVE, 1999).

These injuries are also the most devastating incapacitating syndromes that affect humans because, in addition to their severity and irreversibility, in most cases they cause serious disabilities and require a long and costly rehabilitation programme, which often does not lead to a total improvement in the condition, but to an improvement in the individual's adaptation to their new condition. In this context, rehabilitation seeks to develop the remaining capacities, allowing the individual to achieve independence in physical, professional and social activities, according to their level of injury (GREVE, 1999).

There are now more than two hundred thousand Americans (USA) with spinal cord injuries and approximately more than 10,000 new cases of traumatic injuries every year. This condition is the second most expensive treatment condition in hospitals in the United States, with an annual expenditure of approximately fifty-three thousand dollars per patient, with hospital care fees, as well as other taxes for support services to maintain people with spinal cord injuries (WINSLOW and ROZOSVSKY, 2003).

According to the *National Spinal Cord Injury Statistical Centre* (2001), the cost of caring for people with spinal cord injuries in the United States reaches four million dollars every year. Around 38.5% of all causes of spinal cord injury are due to traffic accidents and 24.5% are caused by acts of violence involving firearms and bladed weapons; the etiology also includes, albeit to a lesser extent, sports accidents, falls and accidents at work. The majority of spinal cord injury victims, around 55%, are between 16 and 30 years old and more than 80% of patients affected by this pathology are men.

In Brazil, according to the demographic census carried out in 2000, there were 955,287 people with paraplegia, tetraplegia or hemiplegia. In the Northeast alone there were 275,527 and in Ceará 48,332 cases (IBGE, 2005).

Although epidemiological data on the occurrence of spinal cord injuries in Brazil is unsatisfactory, in a recent study of 92 patients admitted to the Neurosurgery Department of the Santa Isabel Hospital, by Mello *et al.* (2004), the most prevalent causes of trauma were falls (50%) and traffic accidents (40.2%), with the majority of patients being male (80.4%), compared to 19.5% female.

According to a study carried out by the Rede Sarah de Hospitais de Reabilitação (2005) between 1999 and 2000 at the SARAH-Brasília and SARAH-Salvador hospitals, totalling 1,578 admissions, the majority were young adult males (75.9%). Among the patients whose cause of hospitalisation was a spinal cord injury (695 patients), paraplegia predominated (428 patients -61.6%), with the spinal cord injury classified as complete.

Spinal cord injury causes changes in the individual's body dynamics and abrupt transformations, not only for the person, but also for their family and social environment. This leads them to adopt a different lifestyle to adapt to the new situation. There are many changes: bladder and bowel elimination, skin and soft tissues, joint structures, expression of sexuality, nutritional requirements, as well as interferences in the individual's professional life and consequent economic productivity. Spinal cord injury is a serious disabling neurological syndrome characterised by changes in motor skills, superficial and deep sensitivity and neurovegetative disorders in the body segments located below the injury.

The *American Spinal Injury Association* (2002) states that paraplegia is the term used to describe a reduction or loss of motor and/or sensory function of the thoracic, lumbar or sacral segments, compromising the lower limbs, i.e. paraplegia consists of partial or complete paralysis of the lower extremities and the entire trunk or part of it, as a result of damage to the thoracic or lumbar spinal cord or sacral roots (CARVALHO, 2002). Because the spinal cord is preserved superiorly, the person has significant physical ability potential to become independent in all aspects of personal care and mobility with a wheelchair, ambulation, with or without orthoses, crutches and/or a walking stick (STASS *et al.*, 1998; SOMERS, 1992).

According to Mc Donald and Sadowsky (2002) and Maynard *et al.* (1997), spinal cord injuries are classified into complete and incomplete. In complete injuries there is an absence of motor and sensory function below the level of the injury, while in incomplete injuries there is partial preservation of sensory and/or motor function below the neurological level (MAYNARD, 1996).

The pioneering work of Guttman (1976) pointed to spinal cord injuries as a threatening worldwide problem, which in the following decades could become one of the biggest social problems of disability. The belief in the spinal cord injured person as a healthy and potentially productive individual has led to a marked increase in survival over the last 20 years.

Until 1945, the articles published on the subject were clearly concerned with the diagnosis and treatment of spinal cord injury victims. The biggest change came when a large number of World War II veterans returned home. Although combat injuries caused a relatively smaller percentage of spinal cord injuries, veterans needed rehabilitation centres to improve their health care (OZER, 1988). From that time onwards, health sciences advanced sufficiently to allow the incorporation of effective procedures in the rehabilitation of these patients, also pressurised by the fact that survival was increasing (ZEJDLIK, 1992).

As reported by Faro (1996), rehabilitation from trauma should be early, with the aim of avoiding disabilities or even worsening them, and should be considered as a learning process. It is up to the patient, family and health professionals to share responsibility for the gradual reconstruction of a very different life, and in this process physical care will be the first to be learnt, while adjustment will be a lifelong *continuum*.

Rehabilitation, according to Ring (1994), is a dynamic, succession of creative, progressive and educational acts, whose objectives are aimed at the optimum functional restoration of the individual, their reintegration into the family, the community and society, through maximum independence in the activities of daily living.

Several factors need to be considered, including the presence of multiple ailments, functional independence and autonomy.

Borgneth (2004) emphasises that rehabilitation is the practice of scientific concepts aimed at developing the individual's functionality, with a view to their social inclusion, and that the quality of the social inclusion that the individual achieves is related to their greater or lesser independence, both physically and emotionally, and depends on the conduct of the rehabilitation team. He also points out that people with spinal cord injuries need to be contextualised in their family and social environment.

Kirshblum (2004) warns of the advances that have taken place in recent decades in medicine and the consequent increase in the survival of people who have suffered spinal cord injuries, accompanied by an evolution in their treatment, which is now aimed at minimising disabilities and complications and returning the individual to society.

Concern about the rehabilitation of people with motor and sensory deficits caused by a spinal cord injury has led to the creation of various scales to measure the functional capacity of people with spinal cord injuries, including the *Pulse Profile,* the Katz Index of Independence in Activities of Daily Living, the Barthel Index and the *Functional Independence Measure* (FIM).

Although the MIF is rarely used in Brazil, several studies in other countries have shown the importance and applicability of this scale (INOUYE *et al.*, 2001; STINEMAN *et al.*,1998; SEGAL *et al.,* 1993).

MELO and SOUSA (2005) also report that the use of the FIM Scale is effective for various populations and that it does not only assess people with physical disabilities acquired in adulthood and who have suffered functional losses.

The functional assessment is carried out using the adapted and validated MIF, which measures functional capacity and independence, estimating the degree of difficulty or limitations attributed to each patient. It is applied by a previously trained nurse with a 60-hour basic course. It is administered in two stages: **on admission**, as soon as the patient is admitted or up to 72 hours afterwards, and on **discharge**, usually 72 hours before the patient leaves **hospital.** This behaviour was established at the institution in accordance with the *Uniform Data System for Medical Rehabilitation* (1984).

According to Tan (1998), the FIM is used to quantify the effective gain within a rehabilitation programme, and because it is a standardised instrument and the most widely used within rehabilitation.

In this context, nursing plays a key role, as it provides comprehensive patient care through health promotion, recovery and, especially in the context of rehabilitation, supervision and guidance of comprehensive patient care, always aiming for independence.

Our interest in this subject stems from a professional life spent over thirteen years practising rehabilitation in a world reference centre. Along the way, we have developed a clinical speciality in Neurological Nursing and it is with great satisfaction that we have developed our work in this area, since the representation of the spinal cord as a noble organ and vital faculty of our body is an indicator of full life, of freedom to come and go, and because it is an organ closely linked to quality of life issues.

The assessment of the degree of functional independence in people with paraplegia using the FIM arose precisely from the author's daily observation as a nurse providing care to these patients in the Spinal Cord Injury Sector of the Sarah-Fortaleza Rehabilitation Centre.

We share the view that knowing the presentation of patients with spinal cord injuries in terms of functional independence allows rehabilitation services to structure themselves to meet the demands of this population more efficiently. In addition, according to the literature, rehabilitation interventions are based on the application of specific techniques for each patient with the aim of restoring or acquiring the best level of performance in daily life tasks, even if there are residual disabilities. Riberto *et al* (2005) also point out that functional assessment makes it possible to monitor the patient's progress in their rehabilitation process, helping to refine therapeutic interventions and verify gains until a reduction in the rate of improvement is established.

Evaluating the results of a rehabilitation programme using the FIM makes it possible to work on improving the rehabilitation programme in the future, so that functional goals can be set according to each patient, in order to get them back on their feet as quickly as possible and enable them, within their limitations, to live in family and social life.

In view of the above, in the practice of providing direct care to patients suffering from

spinal cord injury, some questions began to be raised, including: **what results are obtained with the use of FIM in a rehabilitation programme for people with traumatic paraplegia? What factors interfere with these results?**

# CHAPTER 2

# STUDY OBJECTIVES

## 2.1 General Objective

- To assess functional independence in people with traumatic paraplegia undergoing a rehabilitation programme.

## 2.2 Specific objectives

- To assess functional independence using the Functional Independence Measurement Scale (FIM);
- to identify factors associated with spinal cord injury (gender, age, time, level and etiology of injury, classification of injury according to ASIA criteria, length of hospitalisation, schooling and associated complications) with gain in functional independence;
- to see if there is a relationship between the associated factors and the degree of functional independence;
- to see how complications (pressure ulcers, heterotopic ossification, spasticity and neuropathic pain) interfere with functional gain in people with traumatic paraplegia;

# CHAPTER 3

# RESEARCH HYPOTHESES

In the face of rehabilitative practice, some facts are observed that will have to be proven or rejected through the results of this research.

The central hypothesis is that there are gains in the capacity for functional independence after participating in and experiencing the rehabilitation programme. These are factors that interfere with this result:

Male spinal cord injured people achieve greater functional independence compared to females;

The age of people with spinal cord injuries affects their gain in functional independence; young people show greater functional gain;

The length of time since spinal cord injury has a positive effect on functional gain, since people with spinal cord injuries who have been injured for longer have greater functional gain;

The motor level of the spinal cord injury interferes with functional gain in a negative way, as patients with higher levels of injury have lower gains;

The etiology and taxonomy of the injury interfere negatively with gains in functional independence, as patients with complete spinal cord injuries gain less functional independence;

*The* length of hospitalisation interferes negatively with functional gain, as patients with longer hospital stays have lower functional gain;

Schooling, on the other hand, has a positive effect on functional gain, as patients with a higher level of education show greater functional gain;

Ethnicity does not interfere with functional gain, as it does not affect the gain in independence of people with spinal cord injuries;

People with spinal cord injuries who are hospitalised on a full-time basis show greater functional gains than those in day hospitals;

People with spinal cord injuries who are hospitalised with companions show less functional gain, as the companion negatively affects the acquisition of gain; and

Secondary complications (pressure ulcers, heterotopic ossification, spasticity, neuropathic pain) and/or those associated with spinal cord injury (brachial plexus lesions) negatively affect the acquisition of functional independence for people with spinal cord injuries.

# CHAPTER 4

# LITERATURE REVIEW

## 4.1 Spinal Cord Injury

In recent decades, knowledge about caring for people with spinal cord injuries has developed and improved considerably. Even so, this type of injury is still one of the most catastrophic, leading to physical, social, economic, emotional and psychological damage, especially when it occurs in young adults (FREED, 1994).

The oldest available documentation on spinal cord injury is found in the surgical papyrus of Edwin Smith, which is estimated to date from between the 3rd and 25th centuries BC. This document depicts a man with a broken neck, paralysed in all limbs and the words "a disease that should not be treated". This prescription was followed for millennia, mainly due to the lack of understanding of the injury and its manifestations. In the century before the First World War, there were advances in surgical procedures for spinal cord injury, which ushered in a new era for people suffering from the problem (FREED, 1994). Even so, to this day, progress is still minimal in terms of recovery from the injury. The great hope at the moment is stem cells, which have been studied all over the world.

With regard to the incidence and aetiology of spinal cord injuries, Botelho (2001) studied patients who had suffered spinal cord trauma in the northern part of the city of São Paulo between 1969 and 2000. He showed an estimated overall incidence of spinal cord trauma of 22.63 million/year and cervical trauma of 8.6 million/year, with a predominance of falls (29%), while car accidents caused 22% of these. Of the falls, slab falls were the most frequent (7.3), and shallow water diving was the third cause, with just under 15 per cent, and the average age was 35 years and 45 per cent of the sample were under 30 years old.

According to Pereira and Araújo (2005), nowadays, due to the recrudescence of episodes associated with urban violence, such as traffic accidents and firearm attacks, a significant number of citizens around the world face the suffering and limitations caused by traumatic spinal cord injury.

The spinal cord comprises all the neural structures contained within the vertebral canal: the spinal cord, dorsal and ventral roots, spinal nerves and meninges. The spinal cord segments exchange information with other spinal cord segments, with the peripheral nerves and with the brain.

According to the *American Spinal Injury Association* (ASIA), spinal cord injuries can be complete or incomplete and are classified on the *Impairment Scale* (AIS),

– AIS A - complete lesion, with no motor or sensory function below the level of the lesion;

– AIS B - incomplete lesion, without motor function below the level of the lesion, but with preserved sensitivity;

– AIS C - incomplete lesion, with preservation of sensory and motor function below the level of the lesion, but reduced muscle strength (between 1 and 3);
– AIS D - incomplete injury, with preservation of sensory and motor function below the level of the injury, with muscle strength greater than or equal to 3 e;

– AIS E - sensory and motor functions are normal.

It is therefore very important for nurses who care for this clientele to be familiar with this classification (AIS), since it is on this basis that we can understand each person's potential for functional rehabilitation.

## 4.2 Rehabilitation

Rehabilitation is a concept that must involve the entire healthcare system. It must be comprehensive and include prevention and early recognition, including post-discharge. Among the objectives sought through rehabilitation are: increased independence, shorter hospital stays and, above all, improved quality of life (GREVE, 1999).


It is important, when assessing a particular illness, to look not only at its aetiological, pathological and clinical aspects, but also to analyse the full consequences of the illness on the psychosocial reality of the individual and their family. Identifying these disabilities, which is the consequence of the functional or anatomical injury secondary to the trauma or illness, which causes difficulties or even prevents the performance of a certain function, is of paramount importance for rehabilitation. From this moment on, their limitations are known and objectives and goals are set to be achieved, which should be aimed at independence in the preserved capacities, family training, if necessary, and the prevention of sequelae, which determines the effectiveness of the rehabilitation process.

For Delisa *et al* (2002), rehabilitation is the process of helping a person to reach their best physical, psychological and social, vocational and educational potential, compatible with their physiological and anatomical deficits, environmental limitations, desires and life plans; it is actively integrating or reintegrating a person whose capacity is diminished into society.


Also according to Delisa *et al* (2002), each patient is an individual being with their own life story and peculiar characteristics, which can decisively determine the preserved functional and psychosocial capacities to be worked on in their rehabilitation.


Silva et al. (2005), report that physical activity such as swimming effectively improves the physical condition of paraplegics and their functional abilities, leading to gains in functional independence, in terms of the positive effects of its practice on functional independence. They go on to say that there is no doubt that the practice of sport and recreation brings countless benefits to people with spinal cord injuries, reflected in improved performance in activities of daily living, the promotion of physical and social well-being and a reduction in the incidence of clinical complications, and along with advances in medicine, other major developments are taking place, resulting in the production of various adaptations that make the practice of a wide variety of sports increasingly accessible to everyone.

According to Pereira (2002), the patient's participation in the activities of the rehabilitation programme, the perception of physical gains and improvement in the degree of functional independence and living with other patients and family members may be the factors that promote a less threatening assessment of the state s of the injury, mobilising individuals towards adaptation without the risk of accommodation.

Preserved abilities should be worked on by a specialised interdisciplinary team, whose goals are to share common values and objectives, aiming for an individualised biopsychosocial assessment, adding up the individual's previous knowledge of rehabilitation, activities of daily living and practice, social context and work activities. The interdisciplinary team will be able to propose a programme that aims to achieve maximum independence, according to the individual's preserved abilities or family training.

The effectiveness and continuation of the rehabilitation process in everyday life will depend on the combined knowledge and decisions of the interdisciplinary team with the individual and family.

In this context, at the Sarah Network of Rehabilitation Hospitals, the rehabilitation programme is developed by an interdisciplinary team and involves various activities aimed at promoting independence and quality of life for people with paraplegia. These activities include:

- assessing the potential of each patient;
- training in activities of daily living - bathing, dressing, transfers, getting around;
- orientation groups on pathology and prognosis;
- orientation groups for self-care;
- bladder, bowel and sexual re-education groups;
- nutrition group;
- assessment and management of possible complications - neurogenic bladder and bowel, spasticity, heterotopic ossification, neuropathic pain, pressure ulcers;
- promoting satisfactory bladder emptying, mainly through training in clean

intermittent catheterisation;

      - locomotion training (whether in a wheelchair or walking with a walker or cane);

      - training in practical life activities (going to the post office, bank, market, etc.);

      - internal socialisation (with other patients) and external socialisation (*shopping, the* beach, etc.), with the aim of promoting greater social interaction;

      - home visits in order to identify architectural barriers and propose solutions;

      - psychological, pedagogical and social assistance support; and

      - physiotherapy and sports activities (basketball, table tennis, swimming, among others).

Rehabilitation, in this context, means creating ways to get people with spinal cord injuries to live with their abilities, creating adaptations to make them as independent and productive as possible, respecting their reserved capacity and improving their quality of life.

However, in order to carry out all these proposals in the rehabilitation programme, the individual's anamnesis, physical examination and functional assessment must be carried out in an appropriate and detailed manner.

Functional assessment is carried out in order to evaluate personal care and the individual's performance in activities of daily living. To do this, a scale should be used to measure the score, so that the interdisciplinary team can programme the objectives to be achieved for their independence or family training, while observing and highlighting their preserved capacity.

In this context, various methods have emerged in the rehabilitation literature and since 1997 the *Functional Independence* Measure (FIM) has been used in the Sarah Network.

The importance of measuring functional outcomes is emphasised by recognition bodies such as the Commission for the Recognition of Rehabilitation Facilities (CARF), as part of a programme evaluation system. And for the team, this assessment is the return to what was proposed, since it is used on admission, during hospitalisation and on discharge.

The MIF is described below.


## 4.3 Functional Independence Measure


The MIF Scale (Appendix 1) was developed in the 1980s by a US team organised by the American Academy of Physical Medicine and Rehabilitation and the American Congress of Rehabilitation Medicine, with the aim of creating an instrument capable of measuring the degree of independence of disabled patients in performing motor and cognitive tasks, and was validated in 1986.


Christiansen and Ottenbacher (1998) report that in the last decade there has been an extraordinary growth in the use of the MIF Scale, largely due to a growing body of research demonstrating its validity in various neurological patients, such as people victimised by stroke and traumatic brain injury, as well as the creation of a database that includes a large number of rehabilitation cases whose progress and results are documented using this scale.

The translation and validation of the FIM was carried out in Brazil by Riberto *et al.* (2001), based on the original English version of the manual and the Portuguese language version produced in Portugal, and followed the guidelines of the World Health Organisation (WHO). According to the same authors, the process involved a translator and bilingual medical staff who were familiar with the nature of the study, and conceptual rather than strictly literary translation was emphasised. The Portuguese version of the instrument was translated back into English, but no conflicts of interpretation were found, as the initial translation process already included the correction of terms that could be sources of confusion. According to the study, cultural equivalence was carried out with 25 health professionals linked to rehabilitation centres in various Brazilian states, who had received formal training to apply the instrument.


Gowland *et al.* (1993) emphasise the need to apply and use well-constructed, validated and reliable measurement scales to assess the effectiveness of therapeutic interventions.

Other authors, such as Heinemann *et al.* (1993) and Linacre *et al.* (1994), have used the FIM to measure the severity of disability and determine the extent to which disability measures are comparable for patients with different disabilities. These authors report that this scale allows for a quantitative comparison of functional independence measures at different times, which confirms its validity.

Although improving the functional independence of people with paraplegia is a primary goal within a rehabilitation programme, little is done to assess the growth potential and effectiveness of these programmes in the context of rehabilitation. One of the advantages of applying the FIM to patients with traumatic paraplegia is the possibility of setting goals and objectives at the time of their admission to the rehabilitation programme and modifying these objectives and goals according to their progress and effective participation in the programme up to the time of their discharge from hospital.

Assessing the functional capacity of people with traumatic paraplegia gives nurses and other members of the interdisciplinary team a more precise view of the degree of independence of each person with a spinal cord injury. Functional assessment is understood as the designation given to a specific function, the ability to carry out self-care and meet their basic daily needs, i.e. carrying out activities of daily living (ADLs).

For Katz *et al* (1963) and Nery (2001), functional capacity is defined as the degree of preservation of the individual's ability to carry out basic activities of daily living, such as bathing, dressing, hygiene and transfers, continental preservation and feeding, and also to carry out instrumental activities of daily living, such as cooking, tidying the house, telephoning, washing clothes, shopping, looking after household finances and taking medication.

Toledo and Diogo (2003) point out that independence in carrying out the tasks of daily living is of great importance in people's lives, as it involves issues of an emotional, physical and social nature. Regardless of age group, dependency can alter family dynamics and the roles played by its members, interfering in the relationships and well-being of the dependent person and their family members.

The seven-level scale represents the most important differences in independent and dependent behaviour. It reflects the volume of care in terms of the time/energy required to achieve and maintain independence. FIM measures what the person is doing exactly at the time of the assessment.

According to Riberto (2001) and Kawasaki and Cruz (2004), the Functional Independence Measurement Scale (FIM) is a multidimensional instrument that assesses the individual's performance in 18 activities distributed in two large domains: motor and cognitive/social. In the motor domain, the emphasis is on self-care, sphincter control, transfer and locomotion, encompassing 13 activities. The cognitive/social domain comprises the functions of communication and social cognition, with five activities.

According to the Uniform Medical Rehabilitation Information System (UDS), the scale is made up of 6 activity groups and 18 sub-groups, and assesses the patient's ability to care for the body (eating, getting ready, bathing, dressing the upper body, dressing the lower body and toileting); sphincter control (bladder and bowel control); transfer (bed, chair, wheelchair, toilet, bath or shower); locomotion (walking, wheelchair, going up and down a flight of steps); communication (level of comprehension and expression) and social integration (social interaction, problem solving and memory).

These items have a minimum score of 1 and a maximum score of 7. For all the items, the score can range from 18 to 126. For each item, the level that best corresponds to the patient's situation is recorded. We chose to record the lowest score obtained during the assessment, as it corresponds to what the patient normally does effectively, because it means that they haven't mastered the function or are too tired or unmotivated to practise it.

Score 7 represents the patient's complete independence in carrying out activities of daily living and can be categorised into two levels: with help and without help. At the unaided level, we consider complete independence with a score of 7 and a score of 6 as modified independence. For the level with help, modified dependence, a score of 5 is given when the patient carries out activities under supervision and 4 when assistance is minimal (the patient performs 75 per cent or more of the tasks). A score of 3 is considered when assistance is moderate (the patient performs 50 per cent or more of the tasks). Complete dependence is when the patient needs maximum assistance (performs at least 25 per cent of tasks), with 2 being the score assigned. The last level, score 1, is considered when assistance is total, i.e. the patient is unable to perform any activity without help.

The function levels and their scores are described in detail below:

1) **independent** - does not need help from anyone to carry out the activity. Can be:
   a)**complete independence (7)** - all the tasks described are carried out safely, without alteration, without help and in reasonable time; and
   b)**Modified independence (6)** - when there is one or more of these occurrences; such as the use of an auxiliary aid, unreasonable time or safety risk.

2) **dependent** - when a person needs to help with supervision or physical assistance for the patient to perform the task or when the task is not performed. Dependence can be moderate or complete. In the case of moderate dependence, the patient performs 50 per cent or more of the work and the levels of assistance required are:
   a)**supervision or preparation (5)** - when the patient just needs someone by their side, encouraging or suggesting. There is no physical contact, but there may be a need to prepare the materials needed to carry out the activity;

   b)**assistance with minimal contact (4)** - when it is only necessary to touch the patient to help them carry out their tasks, or when the patient does 75 per cent or more of the work; and
   c)**moderate assistance (3)** - when more than just touching is required or when the patient does 50 to 75 per cent of the work.

In the case of complete dependence, the patient does less than 50 per cent of the work. Maximum or total assistance is required, otherwise the activity is not carried out. The levels of assistance required are:

   a)**maximum assistance (2)** - when it is necessary to touch the patient, making a great effort to help and the patient cooperates with less than 50 per cent of the effort, but makes at least 25 per cent;
   b) **total assistance (1)** - the patient does less than 25% of the work.

The 18 subgroups are described below

## 1) Body care

a) **Eating** - described as using the appropriate tools to bring food to the mouth, chewing and swallowing, once the meal has been presented in the usual way, on a table or tray.

b) **Getting ready** - includes oral hygiene, fixing hair, washing face and hands, shaving or putting on make-up.

c) **Bathing** - described as washing the body from the neck down (excluding the back) in the bath, shower or bed (with a sponge).

d) **Dressing the upper body** - includes dressing or undressing above the waist as well as putting on and removing prostheses or orthoses.

e) **Dressing the lower body** - this means dressing from the waist down, as well as putting on and removing prostheses or orthoses when necessary.

f) **Toileting** - involves maintaining perineal hygiene, as well as removing and adjusting clothing before and after using the toilet or comadre/parrot.

## 2) Sphincter control

g) **Bladder control** - described as complete control of the act of urinating and use of the equipment or agents needed to control urine.

h) **Bowel control** - including complete intentional control of bowel movements and the use of equipment and agents necessary for bowel control.

## 3) Transfers

i) **Transferring (bed, chair, wheelchair)** - involves all aspects of transferring to and from bed, chair and wheelchair, as well as standing if walking is the person's usual mode of locomotion.

j)  **Transferring (toilet) -** sitting down and getting up from the toilet.

k)  **Transferring (bath or shower) -** and we assess whether the patient can get in and out of a bath or shower.

### 4)  Locomotion

l)  **Getting around (walking/wheelchair) -** walking (standing) or using a wheelchair (sitting) on a flat surface. If the person uses two modes of locomotion with the same frequency, we indicate both in the assessment.

m) **Stairs** - this assesses whether the patient can go up and down a flight of stairs (2 to 14 steps) at home or in hospital.

### 5)  Communication

n) **Comprehension** - means understanding audio or visual communication (e.g. writing, signs and gestures). The most frequent mode of comprehension (auditory and visual) is assessed and checked.

o) **Expression** - this assesses whether the patient can express language clearly orally or not; it covers intelligible speech or the clear expression of language through writing or a communication device. The most common mode of expression is checked.

### 6)  Social Integration

p) **Social interaction** - verifies that the patient is able to relate to and participate with others in social and therapeutic situations, referring to the person's ability to deal with their own needs in conjunction with the needs of others.

q) **Problem-solving** - this assesses whether the patient is able to solve daily life problems, make reasonable, safe and timely decisions on financial, social and personal matters, initiate activities, following a sequence and applying corrections to solve problems.

r)        **Memory** - the patient's ability to recognise and remember while carrying out everyday activities in an institutional or community context is assessed; it includes the ability to store and retrieve information, particularly verbal and visual information. Functional evidence of memory includes recognising people you meet frequently, memorising routines and carrying out tasks without being reminded. A memory deficit impairs learning as well as task performance.

# CHAPTER 5

# METHODOLOGICAL RESOURCES

## 5.1 Type of Study

This is a cross-sectional quantitative study of a retrospective, descriptive nature. The quantitative approach is used when, having a usable and valid measuring instrument, the aim is to ensure the objectivity and credibility of the findings; in this case, the instruments do not jeopardise human life and the proposed question indicates a concern with quantification, when it is necessary to compare events or when it is desirable to replicate studies. Retrospective studies look for information in documents and records of events that occurred in the more remote past. Descriptive research is characterised by the need to explore an unfamiliar situation, about which more information is needed; it seeks to explore a significant reality, to identify its characteristics, its change or its regularity (POLIT, BECKE HUNGLER, 2004; LEOPARDI *et al.*2001).

Descriptive research also aims to highlight known characteristics or components of a fact, phenomenon or problem, and is usually carried out in the form of surveys or systematic observations. Therefore, this type of study aims to accurately describe the facts or phenomena of a given reality and requires the researcher to provide a series of information about what they want to study, a precise definition of techniques, methods, models and theories that guide the collection and interpretation of data (SANTOS, 1999).

## 5.2  Study site

The research was carried out at the Fortaleza Unit of the SARAH Network of Rehabilitation Hospitals. This was created by Law No. 8,246 of 22 October 1991 and aims to return the tax paid by any citizen by providing them with free, qualified medical care. It has units in the following cities in the country: Brasília, Belo Horizonte, Rio de Janeiro, Salvador, Fortaleza, São Luís and Macapá.

The work programme has the following general objectives:

- to provide qualified public medical services in the field of locomotor system medicine;
- train human resources and promote the production of scientific knowledge;
- produce information in the areas of epidemiology, hospital management, quality control and costs of the services provided; and
-   to carry out educational and preventive actions aimed at reducing the causes of the main pathologies treated by the Network.

The SARAH Network hospitals have been interconnected by telecommunications technology since 1997, and are characterised by the careful integration of their architectural design with the principles of work organisation and the different rehabilitation programmes, defined according to the epidemiological indicators of the region in which each unit is located.

In addition, the Sarah Network adheres to the following philosophical principles:

- **create** - a specialised health centre that understands the human being as the subject of action and not as an object on which techniques are applied;

- **experience** - the medicine of the locomotor system as a set of unified knowledge and techniques aimed at restoring to the physically disabled the universal right to come and go.

- **acting** - in society to prevent disability and deformity, while at the same time combating prejudices about physical disability, because what characterises life is the infinite variation of form that changes over time.

- **defend** - the principle that no person may be discriminated against because they are different from the average in their physical shape or way of carrying out an activity.

- **breaking free:** from technological dependence by utilising the creative potential of our culture, rejecting the passive attitude towards consumerism and imitation.

- **develop**: a critical attitude towards imported models, whether techniques or behaviours.

- **simplify**: techniques and procedures to adapt them to the real needs presented by the economic and cultural contrasts of the regions
simplification is the critical synthesis of more complex systems and processes: "you can't simplify what you don't know".

- **valuing** - innovative initiative and the exchange of experiences in teaching and research, stimulating the creativity of individuals and groups, "the individual is the institution" and everyone is accountable to it, dedicating their lives to it.

- **living** - for health and not surviving illness.

- **Transform** - each person into an agent of their own health.

- **Work**: so that the utopia of this hospital is to educate for health, in such a way that everyone, protected from illness, no longer needs it.

- **The community** - is primarily responsible for this work, the purpose of which is to realise its will. It is therefore everyone's duty to hold this institution to the commitment it has made today.

The Sarah Rehabilitation Centre - Fortaleza was inaugurated in September 2001 to treat patients with physical disabilities resulting from spinal cord or brain injuries. Both paediatric and adult patients are cared for. The wards are collective, with gardens and spaces for various activities. It also has support areas such as swimming pools, a gymnasium for functional therapy, complementary diagnostic examination units, libraries, laboratories and various other facilities.

The Rehabilitation Programme for Patients with Spinal Cord Injury is carried out on all the institution's premises, mainly with activities in the infirmary, functional therapy gymnasium, library classrooms, among other places. The infirmary on the 3rd floor currently has capacity for 27 patients. The programme welcomes people with spinal cord injuries from various cities in Brazil, most of them in the north-east.

In order to achieve its objectives, a joint effort by a team of professionals, patient and family is necessary, because the success of the rehabilitation programme depends on the sum of the efforts of all those directly or indirectly involved in this process.

The interdisciplinary team is made up of nurses, physiotherapists (called functional therapists at Sarah), doctors, psychologists, nutritionists, social workers, pedagogues, physical education teachers and pharmacists, among others. These professionals share common values and objectives. Actions must be synchronised so as to always join forces in setting goals to achieve the proposed objectives.

Nurses are an integral and fundamental part of this process, as they are involved in patient care twenty-four hours a day, providing comprehensive care from admission to the outpatient clinic until discharge, planning nursing care in order to optimise the quality provided, identifying complications, providing care directly to the patient in a holistic way, assisting and supervising activities of daily living, guiding the patient and family to identify signs of complications.

## 5.3 Population and Sample

Information on patients with traumatic spinal cord injuries who entered the Spinal Cord Injury Rehabilitation Programme between 1st January 2002 and 31st December 2005 was selected from the electronic medical records. This period was chosen because the Sarah Rehabilitation Centre was set up in Fortaleza at the end of 2001 and ended in 2005 because the database is closed every six months.

The inclusion criteria for the study were: patients with traumatic paraplegia, because only those with traumatic injuries are subject to the ASIA classification, having undergone an initial rehabilitation programme, i.e. their first hospitalisation for rehabilitation, having stayed on the programme for a minimum of 15 days and a maximum of 90 days and having completed the rehabilitation programme, as established by the *Uniform Data System for Medical Rehabilitation* (1984). This last criterion is necessary because some patients start the rehabilitation programme but it is interrupted due to clinical complications, which means that it is not possible to carry out a final assessment using the FIM, only an initial one.

Spinal cord injury patients who had previously taken part in a rehabilitation programme at other units of the Sarah Network of Rehabilitation Hospitals and patients with an associated diagnosis of traumatic brain injury were excluded.

After initial screening according to these criteria, the sample was made up of the population itself.

The subjects were assessed in terms of their gain on the FIM Scale during the hospitalisation period, i.e. the difference between the FIM at discharge and admission, for each of the 18 items mentioned in the literature review. This difference constituted the dependent variable, dichotomised into its median value.

The independent variables to be considered in this study were: age (in years); gender; time from injury to admission to the rehabilitation programme (years); etiology of the traumatic injury; classification of the injury according to ASIA criteria (complete injury, incomplete injury); level of the injury; length of hospital stay (days), schooling and presence of complications (spasticity, pressure ulcer, heterotopic ossification, neuropathic pain).

## 5.4 Data Collection Instruments

The instrument used was the Functional Independence Measure (Appendix 1), as described in the literature review.

In this study, however, only the items in the motor domain were analysed and the items in the cognitive/social domain were not assessed, since patients with spinal cord injuries, without associated brain trauma, do not normally show alterations in these areas.

The FIM recommends these items precisely because this scale is also used in patients with brain injuries such as Traumatic Brain Injury (TBI) and Stroke.

We chose this scale because the Brazilian version has good cultural equivalence, its reproducibility properties are good and it can be used in our country.

## 5.5  Data Collection Procedure

At Rede Sarah, there is a specific computerised system where all the FIM scores are recorded, both on admission and on discharge. It is from this database that the admission and discharge scores of the research subjects were taken.

Another essential system for collecting information was the electronic medical record, since the research information was retrieved from it, characterising the variables involved. An instrument (Appendix 1) was also created to record this data.

After collection, which we carried out by accessing the patients' medical records and the MIF registration system, a statistician from the unit carried out the necessary correlations.

## 5.6  Data Treatment and Analysis

For the statistical analyses, descriptive analyses of sociodemographic and clinical data were initially carried out, with frequency distribution, as well as the calculation of position and dispersion measures. A 5% significance level was used for inferences.

In order to compare the FIM Scale before and after the rehabilitation programme, we used the paired *Student's t-test,* which compares dependent samples using the means of the data, due to normal distribution, and the *Kolmogorov-Smirnov* normality test.

*Pearson*'s correlation coefficient was used to assess the level of correlation between gain in functional independence and the variables age, length of hospitalisation and time since injury. *Sperman*'s non-parametric coefficient was used for the variables level of education and the ASIA Scale.

The average degree of independence was compared with the etiology of the injury, the level of the injury and ethnicity, using the ANOVA (*Analysis of Variance*) test. *Levene*'s test was used to check the degree of homogeneity of the degree of independence between the groups. When the difference was not significant, the *TuKey* post-test was applied.

The dichotomised categorical variables - day hospital, companion, spasticity, pressure ulcer, neuropathic pain, brachial plexus injury and gender - were compared with the degree of independence and analysed using *Student's t-test* for independent samples.

SPSS (*Statistical Package for the Social Science*) *software,* version 13 for *Windows,* was used to tabulate, analyse and draw up some graphs.

We consider the efficiency index to be the ratio of the difference in earnings between admission and discharge to the number of days hospitalised.

## 5.7 Ethical aspects

The project was submitted to the Scientific and Ethical Committee of the institution where the research was carried out. The ethical aspects were guided by the precepts of Resolution 196/1996 of the Brazilian National Health Council, especially with regard to preserving the fundamental bioethical principles of respect for the individual, autonomy, non-maleficence, beneficence and justice.

# CHAPTER 6

## RESULTS

In this chapter, we will present the findings of the study, in terms of characterising the sample in a table with simple and absolute frequencies and the findings on gains on the FIM scale in terms of maximum and minimum gains.

**Table 1 - Characterisation of the sample studied. Fortaleza - CE, 2006**

| Features | Frequency | % |
|---|---|---|
| **Sex** | | |
| Female | 35 | 15,4 |
| Male | 193 | 84,6 |
| **Ethnicity** | | |
| Yellow | 9 | 3,9 |
| White | 116 | 50,9 |
| Black | 33 | 14,5 |
| Others | 70 | 30,7 |
| **Age group (years)** | | |
| Up to 20 years | 15 | 6,6 |
| > 20 - 31 | 96 | 42,1 |
| > 31 - 42 | 63 | 27,6 |
| > 42 - 52 | 34 | 14,9 |
| > 52 - 65 | 18 | 7,9 |
| > 65 years | 2 | 0,9 |
| **Education** | | |
| Not literate | 15 | 6,6 |
| Incomplete primary education | 107 | 46,9 |
| Complete primary education | 27 | 11,8 |
| Secondary school incomplete | 30 | 13,2 |
| Completed high school | 34 | 14,9 |
| Higher education incomplete | 4 | 1,8 |
| Higher education completed | 11 | 4,8 |
| **ASIA scale** | | |
| "A" | 163 | 71,5 |
| "B" | 23 | 10,1 |
| "C" | 20 | 8,8 |
| "D" | 22 | 9,6 |
| "E" | | |
| **Etiology of the injury** | | |
| Traffic accident | 67 | 29,4 |
| Assault (bladed weapon and others) | 11 | 4,8 |
| Impact by Object | 7 | 3,0 |
| Puncture by Firearm (PAF) | 114 | 50,0 |
| Fall | 29 | 12,8 |
| **Injury Time (months)** | | |
| <= 12 | 70 | 30,7 |
| 12,01 - 24,00 | 42 | 10,4 |
| 24,01 - 36,00 | 24 | 10,5 |
| 36,01- 48,00 | 12 | 5,3 |
| 48,01 - 60 | 12 | 5,3 |
| 60,01+ | 68 | 29,8 |
| **Engine level[1]** | | |
| T1 - T6 | 85 | 37,3 |
| T7 - T12 | 99 | 43,4 |
| Lumbar | 31 | 13,6 |
| Thoracolumbar transition | 13 | 5,7 |
| **Complications [2]** | | |
| Spasticity | 106 | 46,5 |
| Pressure Ulcers | 48 | 21,1 |
| Heterotopic Ossification | 15 | 6,6 |
| Neuropathic Pain | 97 | 42,5 |
| **Hospitalisation time (days)** | | |
| <= 20 | 7 | 3,1 |
| 21 - 27 | 32 | 14,0 |
| 28 - 34 | 112 | 49,1 |
| 35 - 41 | 58 | 25,4 |
| 42 - 48 | 17 | 7,5 |
| 49 + | 2 | 0,9 |
| **Hospitalisation** | | |
| Day Hospital | 7 | 3,1 |
| Full regime | 221 | 96,9 |

| | | |
|---|---|---|
| **Escort** | | |
| Yes | 11 | 4,8 |
| No | 217 | 95,2 |

Source: National Quality Control Centre (CNCQ) - Sarah - Fortaleza - 2006

[1] - Classification used by the author. [2] - A patient can have more than one associated complication.

Table 1 shows that there was a predominance of males (84.6%), white ethnicity (50.9%), aged between 20 and 31 years (42.1%), with incomplete primary education (46.9%), a predominance of complete injuries (71.5%), due to firearm perforation (50%),with a duration of injury of less than 12 months (30.7%), motor level T7-T12 (43.4%), with spasticity being the most cited complication (46.5%), with an average length of stay of 33 days (**Table 2),** and the majority of patients were hospitalised on a full-time basis (96.9%) and without companions (95.2%).

Table 2 - Relation of gain on the MIF scale at admission and discharge. Sarah - Fortaleza, 2006.

| MIF ITEMS | ADMISSION | | | HIGH | | | Gain Medium |
|---|---|---|---|---|---|---|---|
| | Minimum | Maximum | Average | Minimum | Maximum | Average | |
| **Body Care** | | | | | | | |
| Feeding | 5,00 | 7,00 | 6,96 | 7,00 | 7,00 | 7,00 | 0,04 |
| Personal hygiene - toilet | 4,00 | 7,00 | 6,88 | 5,00 | 7,00 | 6,98 | 0,10 |
| Bathing | 1,00 | 7,00 | 5,17 | 3,00 | 7,00 | 6,70 | 1,53 |
| Dressing members superior | 1,00 | 7,00 | 6,59 | 6,00 | 7,00 | 6,97 | 0,38 |
| Dressing members lower | 1,00 | 7,00 | 3,87 | 1,00 | 7,00 | 6,34 | 2,47 |
| Post-care hygiene eliminations | 1,00 | 7,00 | 4,75 | 1,00 | 7,00 | 6,63 | 1,88 |
| **Sphincter control** | | | | | | | |
| Bladder control | 1,00 | 7,00 | 2,66 | 2,00 | 7,00 | 5,84 | 3,18 |
| Bowel control | 1,00 | 7,00 | 3,15 | 1,00 | 7,00 | 5,96 | 2,81 |
| **Transfers** | | | | | | | |
| To and from bed | 1,00 | 7,00 | 4,02 | 1,00 | 7,00 | 6,29 | 2,27 |
| To and from the pot | 1,00 | 7,00 | 3,67 | 1,00 | 7,00 | 6,02 | 2,35 |
| To and from the shower | 1,00 | 7,00 | 3,08 | 1,00 | 7,00 | 4,94 | 1,86 |
| **Locomotion** | | | | | | | |
| Chair Wheels/March | 1,00 | 7,00 | 4,89 | 1,00 | 7,00 | 6,05 | 1,16 |
| Stairs | 1,00 | 6,00 | 1,31 | 1,00 | 7,00 | 1,53 | 0,22 |
| **Total** | | | | | | | |
| **Average length of stay (average)** | | | | | | | **33 days** |
| **General Efficiency Index** | | | | | | | **0.62** points |

Source: National Quality Control Centre (CNCQ) - Sarah - Fortaleza - 2006

At the end of this stage, we will discuss the findings, supported by the literature on the subject.

# CHAPTER 7

## DISCUSSION

The discussion will take place according to the findings, which are presented in graphs and tables, based on the literature on the subject.

The data studied showed that 193 (84.6%) patients were male and 35 (15.4%) were female. This can be explained by the inclusion criteria, which recommended patients with traumatic spinal cord injury, which is more common in males; Vall and Braga (2006), in a study on neuropathic pain secondary to traumatic spinal cord injury, found 29 (90.6%) male patients and only 3 (9.4%) female patients. We can see (Appendix b) that the female patients had a higher average gain than the men, but the difference in gain was not significant (p= 0.690). This study confirms previous studies regarding the predominance of males in spinal cord injuries (FLORES *et al.* 1999), (ARRUDA, 2000), (CARVALHO,2004), (LEITE and FARO, 2006).

In our study, when we analysed the age group, we saw a predominance of 96 (42.1) patients aged between 20 and 31, followed by 63 (27.6%) patients aged between 31 and 42, as shown in Table 1. When we analysed the degree of independence by age group, we found that there was greater functional gain in the age group up to 20 years (**Graph 1**). The average age of hospitalised patients was 32.6 years. These indicators are in line with national and international literature, which shows that the majority of spinal cord injury patients are affected in their most productive phase of life, due to the fact that spinal cord injury affects a young population, as reported by Abreu *et al.* (2003) and Collazo *et al.* (2002) in their study on Respiratory Functional Assessment in Patients with Traumatic Spinal Cord Injury.

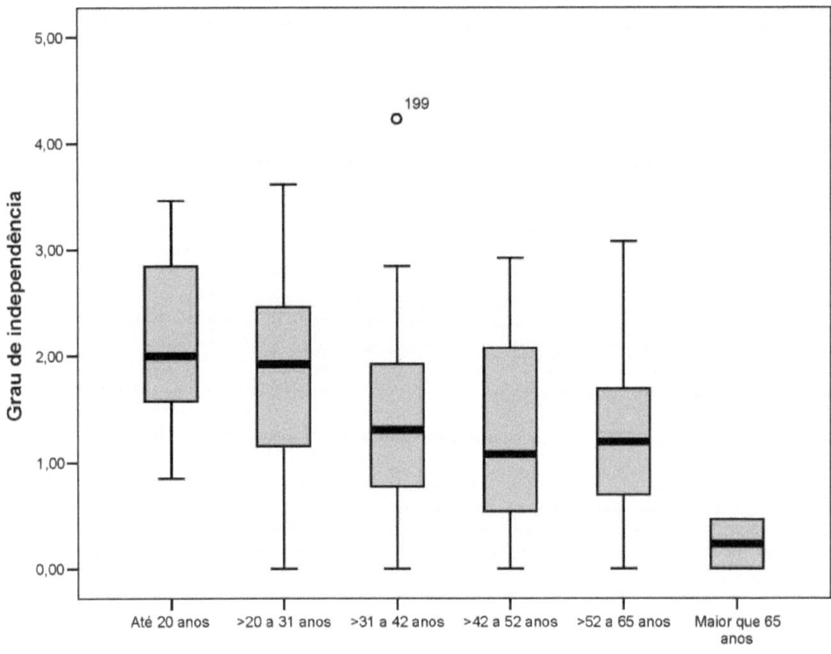


**Graph 1** - Average degree of independence according to **age group of** patients with traumatic spinal cord injury treated at the SARAH Fortaleza hospital - 2006.

Source: National Quality Control Centre (CNCQ) - Sarah - Fortaleza - 2006

As far as the age of the patients is concerned, Arruda (2000), analysing the diagnostic profile of spinal cord trauma patients admitted to the ICU (Intensive Care Unit), points out that the predominant age groups were 15 to 30 years and 31 to 46 years.

According to Defino (1999), spinal cord injury occurs preferentially in males, in a ratio of 4:1, in the 15 to 40 age group, findings corroborated by (Henriques, 2004) and (Pinheiro, 2004).

A study carried out by Bravo *et. al.* (2003) shows that the prevalence of spinal cord injuries in the province of Las Palmas Canarias - Spain is 30.87 cases per 100,000 inhabitants, 44.92 more in men than 16.98 cases per 100,000 inhabitants in women; and the most affected age group is 15-29 years old.

40

In this study, we can see that there is an inverse correlation between the patient's age and the gain (mean on admission - mean on discharge) and that the older the patient, the lower the gain (p < 0.05), as shown in Graph 1.

When we analysed the length of stay, we found that the average length of stay was 33 days. The study in question shows that there is a direct relationship between length of hospitalisation and functional gain; the longer the length of hospitalisation, the greater the functional gain (p< 0.05).

Half of the patients, 114 (50%), had been injured for a maximum of 2 years before being admitted to the rehabilitation programme (**Table 1**). We found that there was an inverse relationship between time since injury and functional gain, as the longer the injury, the lower the functional gain (p< 0.05).

In the opinion of Prandini *et al.* (2002), the rehabilitation programme should begin as early as possible, respecting the clinical conditions of each patient. They also state that the victim of spinal cord trauma goes through various stages, but that the rehabilitation programme can be used at any stage, emphasising the clinical and neurological benefits that can be obtained.

For Mancussi (1998), the period between hospitalisation and the rehabilitation programme, with all the difficulties that come with a spinal cord injury, allows the individual to reflect on the events they have been experiencing. According to the author, the person has returned home in different conditions and will gradually adapt to these new conditions.

Rehabilitation from trauma should be early, with the aim of preventing disabilities or even worsening them. If it is considered a learning process, it is up to the patient, family and health professionals to share responsibility for the gradual reconstruction of a very different life. Adjustment will be a lifelong continuum (FARO, 1996).

According to Sampaio *et al.* (2001) and Henriques (2004), one of the aims of rehabilitation is to help improve self-image, self-confidence and therefore social inclusion.


According to Pereira and Araújo (2005), participation in the rehabilitation programme's activities, the perception of the progressive acquisition of independence, as well as living with other patients and family members may be factors that promote a less threatening assessment of the state of the injury, mobilising individuals to adapt without the risk of accommodation.

Society's view of people with disabilities is drastically altered when they demonstrate independence in their activities of daily living (ADLs), as this goes against the existing social prejudice related to the social and financial burden that people with disabilities have on society. In other words, once they demonstrate independence, the individual has the capacity or potential to exercise their social and productive role in society; physical incapacity turns to independence when people see it that way or when the environment favours it.


In terms of level of education, incomplete primary education predominated, with 107 (46.9%) patients, and secondary education, 34 (14.9%) patients (Table 1). We found that schooling did not interfere with functional gain (p= 0.750) (**Appendix b**).


Graph 2 shows the relationship between schooling and the degree of functional independence.

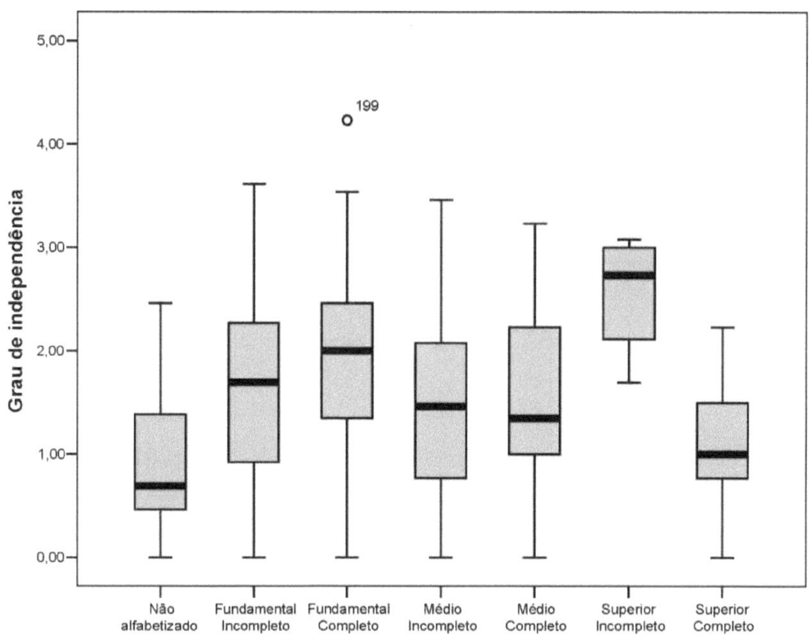


Graph 2 - Average degree of independence, according to the level of **schooling of** patients with traumatic spinal cord injury treated at the SARAH Fortaleza Hospital - 2006.

Source: National Quality Control Centre (CNCQ) - Sarah - Fortaleza

Checking ethnicity (Table 1), we observed a predominance of white ethnicity in 116 (50.9%) of the patients, but this variable did not interfere with functional gain (p=0.982) (**Appendix b**).

With regard to the etiology of the injury, the majority of the 114 patients (50%) were affected by firearm perforation (FAP), followed by road traffic accidents, with 67 patients (29.38%). This etiology was also reported by Vall et *al*. (2005)
who found in their study that the majority of patients were affected by PAF, but this epidemiological profile is different from other regions of Brazil.

A retrospective study of medical records from 2000-2003, carried out by Nogueira (2005) with patients who had suffered traumatic spinal cord injury, showed that the main cause of the injury was PAF, corroborating the data found in our study.

Botelho *et al.* (2001) carried out a study on the epidemiology of cervical spinal cord trauma in the northern zone of the city of São Paulo, between April 1996 and December 2000, and noted that falls were the main cause of spinal cord injury, followed by car accidents.

Traffic accidents stand out among violent deaths, according to Marin and Queiroz (2000), who also point out that they deserve special attention because, as well as deaths, they cause varying degrees of physical disability in a significant number of victims.

Still in relation to aetiology, the majority of patients were affected by firearm perforation (FAP), but there was no significant difference between them (p= 0.075); however, we can see that aggression (white weapon and assault) showed a lower average gain (**Appendix b**).

Penetrating spinal trauma caused by firearms (PAF) is an increasingly prevalent and relevant pathology with a high social and economic cost, due to the sequelae it causes in a generally young population, according to Mery *et al.* (1998), a view we share.

Defino (1999) also says that car accidents, falls from a height, shallow water diving accidents and firearm injuries have been the main causes of spinal trauma. He also reports that the frequency of spinal injuries caused by firearm projectiles has increased considerably, reflecting the high level of violence in large centres.

When we assessed the level of motor lesion, we found 99 (43.4%) patients with a predominance of "low" lesions from T7-T12, followed by "high" thoracic lesions, with 85 (37.3%) patients (Table 1). We found (**Appendix b**) that there was a difference in gain between the level of the lesion and the degree of functional independence (p<0.05). We did, however, observe the formation of 2 groups, thoracic and thoracic-lumbar transition (p<0.05) and that the group of "high" thoracic lesions showed an average gain similar to those of "low" thoracic lesions (1.8271 and 1.6636), respectively. The average gain of the lesions classified as thoracolumbar transition was lower than the lumbar lesion, but when we compared the thoracic lesions with the lumbar and transition lesions, we saw that the gain was higher in the lumbar and transition lesions.

In a study on the functional independence of patients with spinal cord injuries, Riberto *et al.* (2005) observed that patients with thoracic spinal cord injuries had greater functional dependence than those with lumbar spinal cord injuries.

Izquierdo *et. al.* (2002) agree with this statement when they report in a recent study on physical independence in paraplegic patients that paraplegics with spinal cord injuries at the lumbar level have greater functional independence than paraplegics with injuries at the thoracic level. They also emphasise that paraplegic patients are capable of achieving a high degree of independence.

In a retrospective study of surgical cases of traumatic fractures in people with spinal cord injuries between June 1994 and June 2003, Falavigna *et al.* (2005) found 116 cases, predominantly in the thoracolumbar transition (T11-L2), followed by the cervical region and at thoracic level (T1-T10).

Spinal cord injuries at thoracic levels preserve the function of the upper limbs, leaving patients with the potential to become independent in activities of daily living, such as transfers, changes of position, wheelchair management and even driving adapted cars (Ares and Casalis, 2001).

Greve and Castro (2001), on the other hand, observed that when assessing the T6 to T12 level, there is preservation of the upper dorsal extensor muscles, abdominals and paravertebral muscles, so there is greater trunk control. At this level, the patient's main functional goals can be total independence in ADLs, transfer and locomotion in a wheelchair; orthostatism with orthoses; non-functional walking in short environments; no restrictions on driving adapted cars.

Evaluating spinal cord injury according to the *American Spinal Injury Association* (ASIA), we found a predominance of injuries classified as AIS "A", with 163 (71.5%) patients, followed by AIS "B" injuries, with 23 patients (10.1%). The study shows an inverse relationship between the classification of the injury (AIS A, B, C, D or E) and functional gain; the more severe the injury, the greater the functional gain that the spinal cord injury patient acquires (p< 0.05). Although graph 3 shows that people with spinal cord injuries classified as AIS "A" have made more gains in functional independence, we can infer that the person with a spinal cord injury admitted to the rehabilitation programme with greater independence shows less gain than the more dependent institutionalised person.

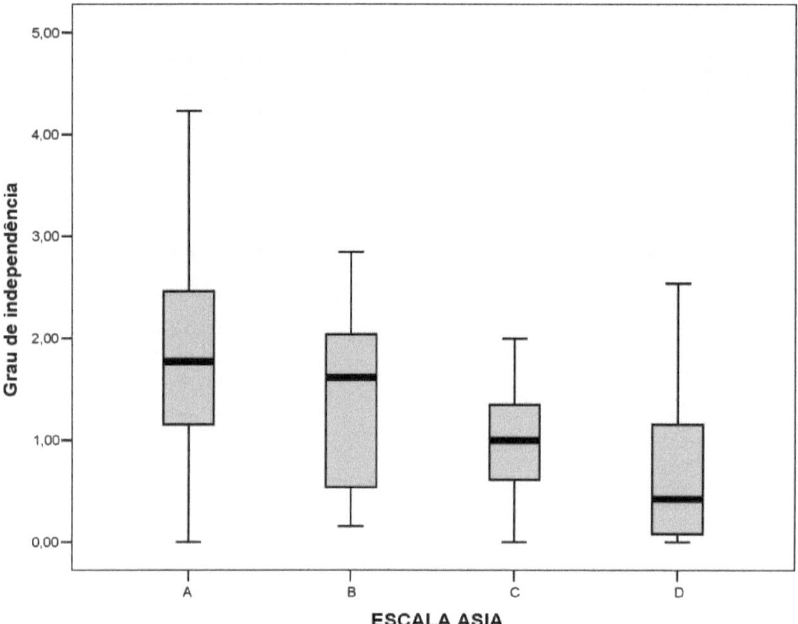


Graph 3 - Average degree of independence according to the **AIS** classification of patients with traumatic spinal cord injury treated at the SARAH Fortaleza hospital in 2006.

Source: National Quality Control Centre (CNCQ) - Sarah - Fortaleza - 2006

Considering the hospitalisation regime, 221 (96.9%) patients were hospitalised 24 hours a day and only 7 (3.1%) patients were in day hospitals (Table 1). With regard to hospitalisation regime, the average gain among inpatients showed no significant differences between 24-hour and day-hospital patients, thus showing that functional gain, using the FIM scale, is independent of hospitalisation regime (p= 0.315) (**Appendix b).

Eleven (4.8%) patients were admitted with a carer. We found that patients admitted with a companion had a higher average gain than those admitted unaccompanied and that the average functional gain of the first group was significant (p< 0.05), the fact that the patient was admitted with a companion had a positive effect on functional gain (**Appendix b**).

According to Carvalho *et al.* (2006), the complexity of specialised care for patients with spinal cord injuries, during hospitalisation and after discharge, means that patients and their families need to receive specific information and training in order to continue this care at home and after discharge.

They also say that, for the family, the teaching shows that they can not only fulfil the role of carer in providing emotional support and comfort and stimulating their family member towards life, but that from now on they are prepared for the continuity of care at home.

Gonzáles *et al.* (2001) state that there is a great need for continuity of care for patients with spinal cord injuries after hospital discharge, and that quality care and preparation for discharge are necessary, including the family in this process, through active participation in the patient's care.

Still on the subject of continuity of care, Carvalho (2004) shows that most of the time, after discharge from hospital, there is a variable period of time for people with spinal cord injuries to join a rehabilitation programme. Therefore, considering the complexity of caring for paraplegics, it is clear that they need to continue receiving specialised care and preparation. The nursing consultation in the outpatient clinic helps in the period between hospital discharge and the rehabilitation programme.

Pereira and Araújo (2005) agree with this statement when they say that clear information and consistent guidance will make it possible to reorganise the life of the person with a spinal cord injury, but also of the members of the socio-family network in which they find themselves, thus contributing to improving the quality of life of everyone involved.

In this sense, Farias *et. al.* (2005) report that it is important to emphasise rehabilitation as an essential factor for patients and their carers, because patients who have had a lesser degree of impairment can acquire greater independence, relieving wear and tear on the carer. They also emphasise the importance of carers in this process.

When we assessed the complications secondary to the spinal cord injury, 106 (46.5%) patients had spasticity; 48 (21.1%) had pressure ulcers; 15 (6.6%) had heterotopic ossification and 97 (42.5%) complained of neuropathic pain (Table 1).

Spasticity is a motor disorder characterised by hypercitability of the stretch reflex with exacerbation of deep reflexes and increased muscle tone (LANCE, 1984), (TEIVE,1988).

According to Braun and Botte (1999), spasticity can arise in clinical situations such as strokes, cerebral palsy, spinal cord injuries, neoplasms, traumatic brain injury, hereditary degenerative and demyelinating diseases, among other alterations of the upper motor neuron.

Heterotopic ossification is a metaplastic biological process in which bone is neoformed in soft tissues adjacent to large joints, where bone tissue is not normally found. It is common not only in patients with spinal cord injuries, but also in those who have suffered cranio-encephalic trauma, severe burns or who have undergone surgical interventions (GREVE E CASTRO, 2003).

According to Hartmann *et al*. (2004), in patients with spinal cord injury, the incidence of heterotopic ossification varies from 13% to 81%, with only 10% to 20% of these patients presenting clinical alterations, which is contrary to our study, where the incidence was 6.6%. The authors also say that the process usually begins in the second month after the trauma, but can start up to a year after the spinal cord injury.

One of the most feared complications of spinal cord injury is heterotopic ossification because it develops asymptomatically and often surprises both the patient and the healthcare team (GREVE and CASTRO, 2003).

Although heterotopic ossification has nothing to do with gaining functional independence, as seen in our study; Castro and Greve (2003), when assessing the prevalence of class I and II human leukocyte antigens (HLA) in patients with traumatic spinal cord injury and their relationship with heterotopic ossification, assessed 57 patients, 28 (52%) of whom had this complication.

When we assessed all the complications (Table 1) in the total sample, i.e. 228 patients, we found that 187 (82.0%) of the patients had some complication secondary to their spinal cord injury (spasticity, pressure ulcers, heterotopic ossification and neuropathic pain).

We observed that whether or not the patient had spasticity did not interfere with functional gain (p= 0.954), just as pressure ulcers do not interfere with functional gain (p= 0.411). When we looked at the complications of heterotopic ossification and neuropathic pain, we also noticed that functional gain depended on these complications (p= 0.657) and p(= 0.868) respectively (**Appendix b**).

Although we found no association between functional gain and the presence of pressure ulcers, pressure ulcers (PUs) are one of the most frequent and serious complications in paraplegics.

According to the *National Pressure Ulcer Advisory Panel* (NPUAP, 1989), a pressure ulcer is defined as a localised area of cell death, developed when soft tissue is compressed between a bony prominence and a hard surface for a prolonged period of time.

Nogueira (2005), in a retrospective study of medical records from 2000-20003 on the occurrence of pressure ulcers in patients suffering from traumatic spinal cord injury, found that the thoracic neurological level was predominant in 44.7% of patients.

A study carried out by Carcinoni *et al.* (2005) in a teaching hospital with 54 patients suffering from traumatic spinal cord injury found that patients with pressure ulcers had a longer hospital stay than those without.

Among the most common complications in people with spinal cord injuries, pressure ulcers have a prevalence of between 25 and 40 per cent (O' CONNOR; KIRSHBLUM, 2001; SOMERS, 2001). The decrease in physical mobility, activity and sensory perception is responsible for the increased risk of a person with a spinal cord injury acquiring a pressure ulcer.

According to Costa and Lopes (2003), patients with spinal cord injuries are more vulnerable to pressure ulcers as they are exposed to a series of internal and external factors responsible for this type of injury.

These authors also report that knowledge of the internal and external factors that predispose to this type of condition is necessary so that, based on these, educational actions can be developed to prevent these ulcers and improve care for individuals already suffering from this type of injury.

In a recent study carried out by Leite and Faro (2006), with the aim of identifying the factors associated with pressure ulcers in paraplegic individuals, related to leisure activities with less movement, pressure ulcers were present in 25 individuals, corresponding to 70% of cases. They also say that a holistic approach on the part of rehabilitation professionals is of fundamental importance for the effectiveness of pressure ulcer prevention in terms of the acceptance and practice of preventive biopsychosocial measures, both for the paraplegic and for rehabilitation professionals in their technical and scientific competence.

According to the *International Association for the Study of Pain* (IASP), "pain is an unpleasant sensory and emotional experience that is associated with actual or potential injury or described in terms of such injury"; it also says that central neuropathic pain after spinal cord injury or myelopathic pain is a consequence of the primary injury or dysfunction of the nervous system.

In this vein, Cordeiro (2005) reports that chronic pain is more frequent in people with spinal cord injuries and can interfere with functional rehabilitation, socio-occupational adaptation and the patient's quality of life.

Various authors have reported that the incidence of pain among spinal cord injury patients has varied from 27% (DAVIS,1975) to 79% (RICHARDS *et al.* 1980, TURNER et *al.*,2001).

Although we found no association between neuropathic pain (p= 0.868) and functional gain, 97 (42.5%) patients had neuropathic pain (**Appendix b**).

This fact is reported by Vall and Braga (2006) in their recent study, which concludes that there is no correlation between pain and the variables gender, age, time of injury, aetiology and neurological level, i.e. neuropathic pain affects individuals with traumatic spinal cord injury regardless of these variables.

Of the total sample evaluated, we found only 4 (1.8%) patients with brachial plexus injury, but in the study, no relationship was found between brachial plexus injury and functional gain (p=0.205), (**Appendix b**).

According to Sedel (1987), the brachial plexus (BP) is a particularly critical region of the peripheral nervous system in terms of its exposure to trauma. And according to Mumenthaler (1969), due to its special anatomical relationship with the mobile structures of the neck and shoulder, it can be involved when force vectors cause traction on these structures

According to Flores (2006), brachial plexus trauma in adults most often results from traction mechanisms on nerve structures, with motorbike accidents being the type of activity most frequently associated with these injuries; this mechanism causes root avulsion in the majority of cases and most patients have some type of injury to other organs or systems. He also says that spontaneous neurological improvement can be observed in 40 per cent of patients and is directly related to the type of trauma mechanism involved.

The gain in the FIM, i.e. the difference between the discharge score and the admission score, divided by the number of days of hospitalisation, shows us the efficiency index, which in our study was 0.62 points (Table 2).

Within the body care group, we found that the item with the greatest gain was dressing the lower limbs, with an average of 3.87 points on admission to 6.34 points on discharge, with an average gain of 2.47 points **(Table 2)**.

Although we haven't looked at the variables that led patients to make greater gains in body care, we can see from the daily care provided that there are numerous variables that interfere with this gain, ranging from the motor level of the injury to the functional adaptations made in the place where daily body hygiene takes place. As a rule, the environmental arrangements were not carried out at home, which meant that the patient gained significant independence when he mastered how to handle them. There were functional gains in all categories.

Within this same group, we found that the post-elimination hygiene item went from an average gain on admission of 4.75 to an average gain of 6.63 points on hospital discharge, with an average gain of 1.88 points.

We can also see that in the body care group, the item with the least functional gain was feeding, with an average of 6.96 points during hospitalisation and an average of 7.0 points at discharge, with an average gain of 0.04. This can be explained by the fact that most patients had a predominance of "low" T7-T12 lesions, with 99 (43.4%) patients, and by the high average level of independence during hospitalisation. Graph 4 shows the average gain on the MIF Scale in all groups.

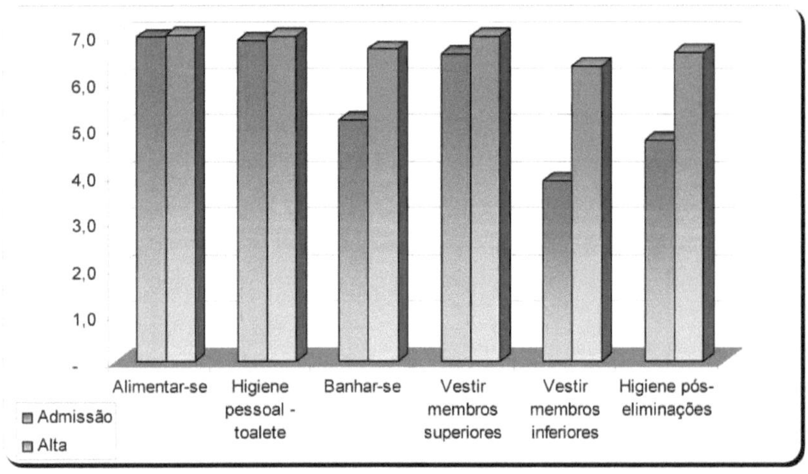


Graph 4 - Average gain on the MIF scale in **body care for** patients with traumatic spinal cord injury treated at the SARAH Fortaleza hospital - 2006.

Source: National Quality Control Centre (CNCQ) - Sarah - Fortaleza - 2006

When we analysed the functional gain in the MIF Scale items related to the average length of hospital stay, we found that the item with the highest average gain was sphincter control, specifically in the bladder control score, which went from an average of 2.66 on admission to 5.84 on discharge. We found an average gain of 3.18 points, followed by bowel control, which went from an average of 3.15 on admission to 5.96, with an average gain of 2.81 points. From the rehabilitation practice, we can infer that this gain may have been influenced by the acquisition of knowledge about bladder care through the bladder reeducation class, the institution of the intermittent catheterisation programme, in most cases the bladder reeducation classes and daily learning on the ward about bladder care.

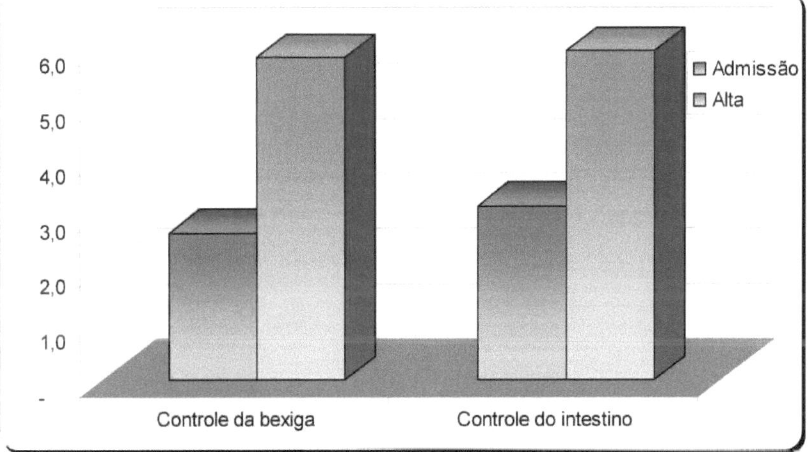


Graph 5 - Average MIF scale score for **sphincter control in** patients with traumatic spinal cord injury treated at the SARAH Fortaleza hospital - 2006.

Source: National Quality Control Centre (CNCQ) - Sarah - Fortaleza - 2006

Within the transfers group, the biggest average gain was 2.35 in relation to transfers from the wheelchair to the pot and vice versa, as the average on admission was 3.67 points and on discharge 6.02 points; followed by the transfer from the wheelchair to the bed and vice versa, from the average on admission of 4.02 points to the average on discharge of 6.29 points, with an average gain of 2.27 points.

When it came to transferring from the wheelchair to the bed, toilet or shower, rehabilitation also gave patients functional gains.

We can try to relate this gain to the patient's general condition, the participation of the family and/or carer during their rehabilitation, motivation and also the mechanisms used to facilitate their activities of daily living, such as: adaptations in the bathroom, the model of bed used in the institution, the model of wheelchair, the balance triangle and trunk balance.

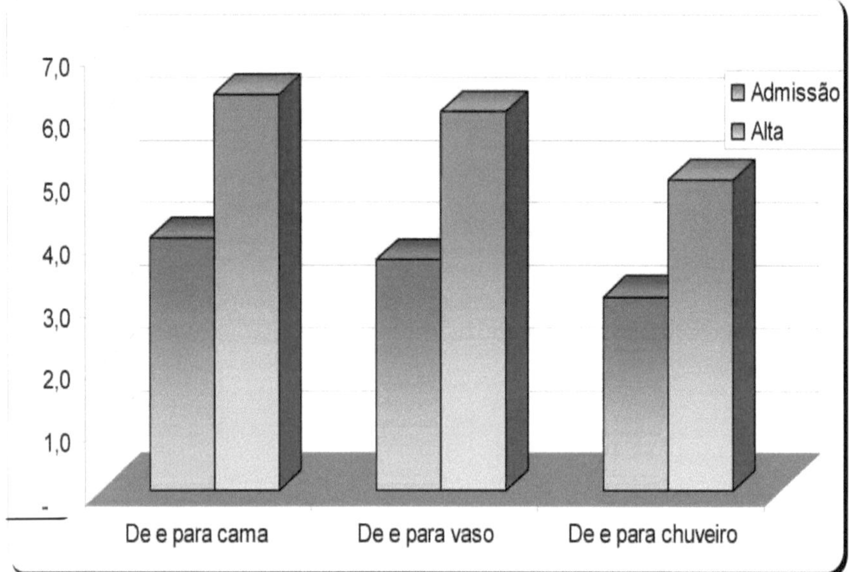


Graph 6 - Average score on the MIF scale for **transfers of** patients with traumatic spinal cord injury treated at the SARAH Fortaleza hospital - 2006.

Source: National Quality Control Centre (CNCQ) - Sarah - Fortaleza - 2006

Evaluating the locomotion group, we found that the greatest gain was in wheelchair/walker locomotion, with an average of 4.89 on admission to 6.05 on discharge, with an average gain of 1.16 points.

We have to consider that the majority had "high" thoracic paraplegia, and most of the time it preserves the function of the upper limbs, leaving them with the potential to become independent in activities of daily living, such as transfers, changes of position, wheelchair management and even driving adapted cars.

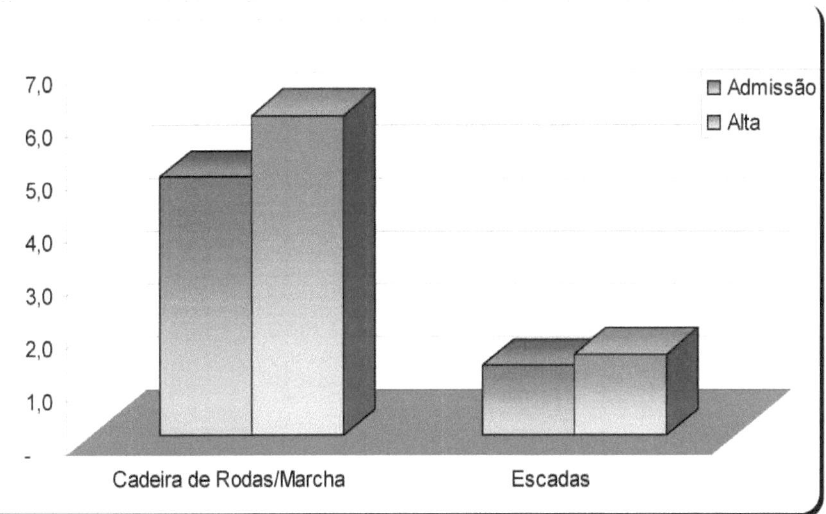


Graph 7 - Average degree of **locomotion on** the MIF scale for patients with traumatic spinal cord injury treated at the SARAH Fortaleza hospital - 2006.

Source: National Quality Control Centre (CNCQ) - Sarah - Fortaleza - 2006

# CHAPTER 8

## CONCLUSIONS

According to the central hypothesis of the research, we concluded that there are gains in functional independence capacity after participating in and experiencing the rehabilitation programme, but we found that some hypotheses were refuted.

Compared to the initial hypotheses, we can say that they influence functional gain:

Age influences functional gain; the younger the person with a spinal cord injury, the greater the functional gain;

The time since the injury interferes with functional gain; the older the injury, the lower the functional gain;

Motor level interferes with functional gain, since "high" injuries gain less than "low" injuries;

There is an inverse relationship between the classification of the injury (AIS; A, B, C, D or E) and functional gain; the more disabling the injury, the more functional gain the patient acquires;

J that there is a direct relationship between length of hospitalisation and functional gain; the longer the length of hospitalisation, the greater the functional gain; and

The person with an internal spinal cord injury who is accompanied by a carer has a greater functional gain.

In our study, gender, aetiology, schooling and ethnicity did not influence functional gain.

We also saw that functional gain using the MIF scale is independent of the hospitalisation regime; and secondary complications (spasticity, heterotopic ossification, pressure ulcers and neuropathic pain) and/or those associated (brachial plexus injury) with spinal cord injury do not interfere with functional gain.


Traumatic spinal cord injury most often occurs abruptly, causing the person and their family to change their lifestyle, especially with regard to their most fundamental right, which is to come and go, as it affects their mobility as well as their sensitivity.


It can also lead to a series of complications typical of spinal cord injury, such as pressure ulcers, spasticity, heterotopic ossification and neuropathic pain, among others.


In addition to the clinical complications, people with spinal cord injuries often suffer from associated depression, as they are suddenly dependent on a family member or carer to provide the most basic care, depending on the level and classification of their spinal cord injury.


The readaptation of people with spinal cord injuries to their new living conditions depends on how they view their "new life", and above all on their initial rehabilitation, which must begin with and be conducted by a multi-professional team, so as to restore the spinal cord injured person to their full functional capacity, according to their potential, reintegrating them into their community as quickly as possible.

Nursing, through the intermediary of nurses, plays a fundamental role in the rehabilitation of people with spinal cord injuries, as it provides nursing care in a holistic manner, enabling people with spinal cord injuries to develop their residual abilities.


Considering the complexity of people with spinal cord injuries, we realised that our study has some limitations, among which we can highlight the following:


- a study based on electronic medical records, where information can sometimes be underreported;

- a shortage of articles, both national and international, on the subject under study;

- the study did not address socio-environmental variables, such as housing conditions, accessibility, sanitary conditions, family income, social support network, among others; and

- The study was carried out in a single rehabilitation centre, causing a sample bias, as the sample studied consisted only of the clients who took part in the rehabilitation programme at this centre.

As suggestions for further studies, we would emphasise the importance of carrying out quantitative studies with clients from other institutions that treat people with spinal cord injuries in the acute phase of the injury, as well as qualitative studies in which we can assess the understanding and feelings of people with traumatic paraplegia in the face of their spinal cord injury.

## REFERENCES

ABREU, M.M, LIMA, J.M.B,FIGUEIRÓ,R.F.S. Mortality and morbidity due to traffic accidents - a contribution to the study of spinal cord injuries. **Escola Anna Nery Revista de Enfermagem**, Rio de Janeiro, v.7, n.1, p.97-103, April, 2003.

AMERICAN SPINAL INJURY ASSOCIATION INTERNATIONAL (ASIA); Medical Society of Paraplegia. **International standards for neurological classification of spinal** cord injury, 2002.

ARES, M.J.J.;CASALIS,M.E.P. Evaluation of disability and functional levels. In: Greve, J.M.D.;CASALIS,M.E.P.; BARROS FILHO,T.E.P. **Diagnóstico e tratamento da lesão da medula espinhal**. São Paulo: Roca, 2001. p. 87-92.

ARRUDA, A.J.C.G. Nursing diagnostic profile of trauma patients admitted to the ICU, in the light of Roy's reference. João Pessoa: Master's dissertation. **Department of Nursing, Federal University of Paraíba** (Univ. Fed. Da Paraíba), 2000.

BOTELHO, R.V. *et al.* Epidemiology of cervical spinal cord trauma in the northern zone of the city of São Paulo. **Arq.Bras.Neurocir**. São Paulo, 20 (3-4): 64-76, 2001.

BORGNETH, L. Considerations on the rehabilitation process. **Acta Fisiátrica**, São Paulo, 11(2); 55- 59, 2004.

BRAUN,R.M.,BOTTE, M.J. Treatment of shoulder deformity in acquired spasticity. **Clin Orthop**. 1999; 368:54-65.

BRAVO, A.M.G. *et.al.* Epidemiology of spinal cord injury in the province of Las Palmas . **Rehabilitación**, Spain, v.37 n°02,p.86-92,marzo 2003.

CARCINONI,M.,CALIRI,M.H.L,NASCIMENTO,M. S. Occurrence of pressure ulcers in individuals with spinal cord injuries. **REME**, Belo Horizonte, v.9, n.1,p.29- 34,2005.

CARVALHO, Z. M.de F. Nursing care for hospitalised paraplegics: a study in the light of Jean Watson's theory of transpersonal care. Fortaleza: Doctoral thesis. **Department of Nursing, Faculty of Pharmacy, Dentistry and Nursing, Federal University of Ceará** (Univ. Fed. do Ceará), 2002.

CARVALHO,Z.M.de F. Faith-hope: nursing diagnoses and interventions. **Enfermeria Integral**, Valencia, n.67, p: XXIV to XXIX, 2004.

CARVALHO,Z..M.de F. O cuidado de enfermagem dirigido as pessoas com lesão vértebro-medular. **Interações**,Coimbra n.6, p.p.175-183., 2004

CARVALHO,Z..M.de F. *et. al.* Patients with spinal cord injury: teaching experience about care for their families. **Escola Anna Nery Revista de Enfermagem** , Rio de Janeiro, v. 10, n.02, p.316-22,agosto 2006 .

CHRISTIANSEN, C.H, OTTENBACHER, KJ. Evaluation and management of daily self-care requirements. **In: DELISA JA**, editor. Rehabilitation medicine: principles and practice. 3ᵃ d ed. Philadelphia: Lippincott Williams & Wilkins; p.137-65, 1998.

COLLAZO, Á.H. *et al* - Thoracic and lumbar spinal cord trauma. **Rev. Cubana Ortopedia Traumatología**. Ciudad de la Habana, 16 (1-2): 53-60, 2002.

COSTA, J.N, M.V.O.LOPES. Review of pressure ulcers in patients with spinal cord injury. **Rev.RENE**. Fortaleza, v.4,n.1,p.109-115,jan./jun.2003.

CORDEIRO, I. F. Conservative versus surgical treatment of traumatic paraplegia due to thoracic and lumbar vertebral fractures. Valencia: Doctoral thesis. **Department of Medicine** (Universitat de Valéncia - Spain), 2005.

DAVIS, R. Pain and suffering following spinal cord injury. **Clin Orthop**. 112 (76-80), 1975.

DEFINO, H.L.A. Trauma to the spinal cord. **Medicina**, Ribeirão Preto, 32:388-400, Oct.-Dec. 1999.

DELISA, JA. *et al*. **Treatise on rehabilitation medicine:** principles and practice. 3rd ed. São Paulo: Manole, 2002.

FALAVIGNA, Asdrubal *et al* . Traumatic fracture of the thoracic spine T1-T10. **Arq. Neuro-Psiquiatr.**, São Paulo, v. 62, n. 4, 2004.

FARIAS,H.H.Q. *et.al*. Being a Carer of an Elderly Person with a Brain Injury: A Theoretical Study. **Rev.REME**, Fortaleza,v.6,n.3,p.112-119,2005.

FARO, A.C.M. and Nursing care for patients with spinal cord injury. In:VENTURA, M. de F. et al. **Enfermagem Ortopédica**. São Paulo: Ícone, 1996. p.175-89.

FREED, M.M. Traumatic and congenital spinal cord injuries. In: KOTTKE, F.J; LEHMANN, J.F. **Krusen's Treatise on Physical Medicine and Rehabilitation**. 4 ed., vol. 2. São Paulo: Manole, 1994.

FLORES, Leandro Pretto *et al*. Prognostic factors of spinal cord trauma caused by firearm projectiles in patients submitted to laminectomy. **Arq. Neuro- Psiquiatrica**, São Paulo, v. 57, n. 3B, 1999.

FLORES, Leandro Pretto. Epidemiological study of the traumatic brachial plexus injuries in adults. **Arq. Neuro-Psiquiatr.**, São Paulo, v. 64, n. 1, 2006

GONZALES, R.C.I , VILLA, T.C.S, CALIRI,M,H,L. The care process for patients with spinal cord injury: case management as a strategy for organising hospital discharge. **Medicina**, Ribeirão Preto, vol.34, p.325-333,jul./dez., 2001.

GREVE J.M.D. Rehabilitation in spinal cord injury. **Rev. Med** 1999; 78 (2): p.276 - 286.

GREVE,J.M.D.;CASTRO,A.W. Locomotion in spinal cord injury. In: Greve,J.M.D.;Casalis, M.E.P.; Barros Filho, T.E.P. **Diagnosis and treatment of spinal cord injury**. São Paulo: roca, 2001, p. 75-79.

GREVE,J.M.D.;CASTRO,A.W. Heterotopic ossification in patients with traumatic spinal cord injury: association with HLA system antigens. **Acta Ortopédica Brasileira**. 11(2), p.102-109 , São Paulo, April-June, 2003.

GUTTMAN L. **Spinal Cord Injuries**. Comprehensive Management and Research. 2nd ed.(UK):Blsckwell Scientific Publications: 1976.

GOWLAND, C.; *et al*. Measuring physical impairment and disability with the Chedoke-McMaster stroke assessment. **Stroke**, v. 24, p. 58-63, 1993.

HARTMANN, Ana P.B.J.; *et al*. Diagnostic imaging in the evaluation of heterotopic ossification. **Rev.Bras. Reumatol**. São Paulo, v.44,n.4,p.291-3, jul/ago,2004.

HENRIQUESA, F.M.D. **Paraplegia, paths of adaptation and quality of life**. Coimbra: Formação e Saúde Ltda. 2004

HEINEMANN et al. Relationships betwee impairment and physical dysabulity as measured by the functional independence measure. **Arch.Phys. Med**.Rehabil.,v.74,p.566-73, 1993.

IBGE. Brazilian Institute of Geography and Statistics. Ministry of Planning, Budget and Management, **Available at: http://www.ibge.gov.br.Acesso, on 31 May 2005.**

INOUYE M, HASHIMOTO H, MIO T, SUMINO K. Influence of admission functional status on functional change after stroke rehabilitation. **Am J Phys Med Rehabil** 2001; 80: 121-5.

IZQUIERDO A.R.T. *et.al.*     Physical Independence in Paraplegic Patients . **Rehabilitación**, Spain, v.36 n°03,p.155-161,miércoles/mayo 2002.

KATZ, S, *et al.* Studies of illness in the aged. The Index of ADL: a standardised measure of biological and psychosocial function. **JAMA** 1963;185:914-9.

KAWASAKI, K; CRUZ, k.C.T. A utilização da medida de independência funcional (MIF) em idosos; uma revisão bibliográfica. **Med.Reabil**; São Paulo; 23(3): 57-60, Sep.-Dec.2004

KIRSHBLUM. S. New rehabilitation interventions in spinal cord injury. **J Spinal Cord Med** 2004; 27:342-50 [ **Medline** ].

LEOPARDI, Maria Tereza. *et al.* **Metodologia da Pesquisa em Saúde**. Santa Maria: Pallotti, 2001.

LEITE, V.B.E, FARO, A.C.M. identificação de fatores associados às úlceras por pressão em indivíduos paraplégicos relacionados às atividades de lazer. **Acta Fisiátrica**, São Paulo, vol 13 (1): 21-25, 2006.

LIANZA, Sergio. **Rehabilitation Medicine**. 3 ed. Rio de Janeiro: Guanabara Koogan, 2001.

LINACRE *et al.* The structure and stability of the functional independence measure. **Arch.Phys. Med.Rehabil.** v.75, p.127-32, 1994.

MANCUSSI, Ana Cristina. Assistance to the patient/family binomial in the situation of traumatic spinal cord injury. **Rev. Latino-Am. Enfermagem**, Ribeirão Preto, v. 6, n. 4, 1998.

MARIN,L.; QUEIROZ, M.S. A actualidade dos accidentenets de trânsito na era da velocidade: uma visão geral. **Caderno de Saúde Pública**, Rio de Janeiro, v.16, n.1, p.7-21, jan/mar 2000.

MAYNARD JÚNIOR, F.M. International standards for neurological and functional classification of spinal cord injuries. Portuguese edition 1999 by Tarcisio EP Barros Filho. **American Spinal Injury Association International**, 1996.

MAYNARD JÚNIOR F.M. *et al.* International standards for neurological and functional classification of spinal cord injury. **Spinal Cord** 1997; 35: 266 - 274.

MELO, Débora Couto; SOUSA, Renata Marinho de. Functional assessment of adult ADEFU users who developed the injury in childhood or have congenital alterations using the Functional Independence Measure (FIM). In: SIMPÓSIO INTERNACIONAL DO ADOLESCENTE, 2., 2005, São Paulo.

Mc DONALD J.W., SADOWSKY C. Spinal Cord Injury. **The Lancet** 2002; 359: 417425.

MELLO, L.R *et al.* Spinal cord injury. Prospective study of 92 cases. **Arq.Bras.Neurocir.** São Paulo, 23 (4): 151-146, 2004.

MERY, Francisco *et al.* Penetrating spinal trauma by firearm. **Rev. chil. neuro-psiquiatr.** Santiago de Chile, Jul.-Sept.1998; 36(3), p.189-193.

MUMENTHALER M. Some clinical aspects of peripheral nerve lesions. **Eur Neurol**; 2:257-268, 1969.
[ Medline]

NATIONAL SPINAL CORD INJURY STATISTICAL CENTER, Facts and Figures at a Glance, May 2001, Available at: **http: spinalcord.uab.edu, accessed on 31 July 2005.**

**NATIONAL PRESSURE ULCER ADVISORY PANEL.** Pressure Ulcer prevalence, cost and risk assessment: concensus development conference statement. **Decubitus**, v.2, n.2,p.24-28, 1989.

NERY AL. **Keywords in Gerontology**. São Paulo: Alínea; 2001.

NOGUEIRA, P. C. Occurrence of pressure ulcers in hospitalised patients with traumatic spinal cord injury: Master's thesis. **Ribeirão Preto Nursing School** - University of São Paulo/USP, 2005.

O'CONNOR,K.C.;KIRSHBLUM,S.C. Pressure ulcers. In: DELISA, J.A;GANS,B.M. **Tratado de Medicina de reabilitação**: princípios e prática. 3.ed.Rio de Janeiro: Manole, 2001, p.1113-1128.

OZER M.N. The management of persons with spinal cord injury. In:      Principles      of spinal cord injury management. New York: **Demos**, 1988:1-11.

PEREIRA, M.E.M.S. Aspectos psicológicos da reabilitação em traumatismo spinalimedular: modalidades de enfrentamento do paciente e seu familiar/acompanompanhante. Brasília: **Master's dissertation. Institute of Psychology, University of Brasília** (Univ. de Brasília), 2002.

PEREIRA, M.E.M.S; ARAÚJO,T.C.C.F. Coping strategies in the rehabilitation of spinal cord injury. **Arq.Neuro-Psiquiatr.**, São Paulo, v.63 n.2b, p.502- 507, jun. 2005.

PINHEIRO,J.P. *et. al.* **Wheelchair**: from the clinic to the user. Coimbra: Quarteto. 2004.

POLIT, D. F; BECK, C.T.; HUNGLER, B.P. **Fundamentals of nursing research** - methods, evaluation and utilisation. 5ᵉᵈ . Porto Alegre: Artmed. 2004.

PRANDINI. M.N, FERNANDES,M.R, TELLA Jr.O.I. A reabilitação no paciente com lesão medular por traumatismo raquimedular. **Rev.Bras.Neurologia**, São Paulo, v.38 (2/3), p.06-11, 2002.

SARAH NETWORK OF REHABILITATION HOSPITALS. **Available at: http://www.sarah.br accessed on 03 January 2006.**

RIBERTO, M. *et al* - Reproducibility of the Brazilian version of the Functional Independence Measure. **Acta Fisiátrica**, São Paulo, 8(1); 45-52, 2001.

RIBERTO, M. et al. Functional independence of patients with spinal cord injury. **Acta Fisiátrica.** São Paulo,12 (2): 61-66, 2005.

RICHARDS, J.S. *et al.* - Psycho-social aspects of chronic pain in spinal cord injury. **Pain.** 8(3), 355-66, 1980.

RING, H. - Rehabilitation in the elderly. In: PAHO. **Care for the elderly:** a challenge for the 1990s. Washington (WC): Elias Anzola Pérez; 1994. p.279-88.

SAMPAIO, I. C. S. *et al.* Sports activity in rehabilitation. In: Greve, J. M. D.; CASALIS, M. E. P.; BARROS , T. E. P. **Diagnosis and treatment of spinal cord injury.** São Paulo: Roca, 2001. p. 211-234.

SANTOS, Raimundo dos. **Scientific Methodology:** the construction of knowledge. Rio de Janeiro: DP&L, 1999.

SEDEL L. Management of supraclavicular lesions: clinical examination, surgical procedures and results. **In TERZIS J** (ed). **Microreconstruction of nerve injuries. Philadelphia**: WB Saunders, P.385-392,1987.

SEGAL,M.E.; DITUNNO, J.F.; STASS, W.E - Interinstitutional agreement of individual Functional Independence Measure (FIM) items measured at two sites on one sample of SCI patients. **Paraplegia**, 31: 622-31; 1993.

SILVA, M.C.R.; OLIVEIRA,R.J.; CONCEICAO, M.I.G.. Effects of swimming on the functional independence of patients with spinal cord injury. **Rev Bras Med Esporte**, jul./ago. 2005, vol.11, no.4, p.251-256. ISSN 1517-8692.

SPINAL CORD INJURY. Available on the Internet. **http:||www.spinalcord.uab.edu [17 December 2005 ].**

SOMERS MF. Spinal cord injury: functional rehabilitation. In _________ **Spinal Cord Injuries**. NorwalK: Appleton & Lange, 1992. p. 22-26.

SOMERS,M.F. **Spinal cord injury**: functional rehabilitation. 2nd ed. New Jersey: prentice Hall, 2001. 458p.

STAAS JR., W. F. _et al._ Spinal cord injury and spinal cord medicine. **In: DELISA, J.** A.; GANS, B. M. (ed.). **Rehabilitation Medicine**: principles and practice. 3. ed. Philadelphia : Lippincott-Raven, 1998.

STINEMAN, M.G.; FIDLER, R.C.; GRANGER, C.V.; MAISLING, G. Functional task benchmarks for stroke rehabilitation. **Arch Phys Med Rehabil**, 79: 497-504, 1998.

TAN, J.C. **Practical manual of physical medicine and rehabilitation:** diagnostics, therapeutics, and basic problems. St. Louis : Mosby, 1998.

TOLEDO, E.H; M.J.D. DIOGO, Elderly people with oncohaematological disorders: actions and difficulties in self-care at the beginning of the disease. **Rev. Latino-Am. Enfermagem**,

Nov./Dec. 2003, vol.11, no.6, p.707-712.

TURNER J.A. *et al.* Chronic pain associated with spinal cord injuries: a community survey. **Phys Med and Rehabil** 2001; 82(4): 501-08.

**UNIFORM DATA SYSTEM FOR MEDICAL REHABILITATION**. Functional Independence Measure - FIM. State University of New York: Buffalo, 1984.

VALL, J. , BRAGA.V.A.B, A.P.C. Central neuropathic pain: characteristics and impact on the life of people with traumatic spinal cord injury. **Rev.Dor.** Oct/Nov/Dec 2005, 6 (4), 657-665.

VALL, J. , BRAGA.V.A.B. **Neuropathic pain secondary to spinal cord injury**: quality of life and rehabilitation. Editora Prontuário, 114p, Curitiba, 2006.

WINSLOW, C.; ROZOSVSKY, J. Effect of spinal cord injury on the respiratory system. **Am J Phys Med Rehabil**, V.82, p.803-814, 2003.

ZEJDLIK CP. Management of spinal cord injury. In: _________ . **Health care concepts and spinal cord injury**. 2nd ed. Boston: Jones and Bartlett, 1992:20-27.

# ANNEXES

## Annex 1 Inpatient assessment sheet - "MIF"

# "END"

### INPATIENT ASSESSMENT SHEET

**PACIENTE EM REABILITAÇÃO**

1. NOME _________________________________________________ 2. PRONTUÁRIO _____________

3. DATA DO NASCIMENTO ____ / ____ / ________    4. SEXO ☐    5. ETNIA ☐
                                                        1. Fem   2. Masc        1. Branco   2. Negro

6. ESTADO CIVIL ☐                                                3.Amarelo 4. Índio 5. Outros
   1. Solteiro  2. Casado  3. Viúvo  4. Separado  5. Divorciado

7. ENDEREÇO _________________________________________________________
_________________________________________________________
_________________________________________________________

**DATAS**

9. ADMISSÃO ____ / ____ / ________        10.TIPO DE ADMISSÃO ☐
                                            1. Reabilitação.Inicial   2. Estadia Curta   3. Readmissão
                                            4. Treino Familiar

11 ALTA ____ / ____ / ________        12. PROGRAMA INTERROMPIDO ? ☐
                                            1. Sim   2. Não
                                            (Verificar se o programa foi interrompido e registrar a seguir as datas)

13. DATAS DE INTERRUPÇÃO DO PROGRAMA:

   1 ª Interrupção      a. Data da Transferência        b. Data do Retorno
                          ____ / ____ / ________         ____ / ____ / ________

   2 ª Interrupção      a. Data da Transferência        b. Data do Retorno
                            ____ / ____ / ________         ____ / ____ / ________

   3 ª Interrupção      a. Data da Transferência        b. Data do Retorno
                            ____ / ____ / ________         ____ / ____ / ________

(AS PERGUNTAS 14 A 16 REFEREM-SE A ENCARGOS FINANCEIROS E SEGURO DE SAÚDE)

**DIAGNÓSTICO**

17. GRUPO DE INCAPACIDADE _________    18. DATA DO INÍCIO ____ / ____ / ________
    (Verificar na apostila de treinamento)

19. DIAGNÓSTICO ETIOLÓGICO _________    20. ESCALA ASIA (apenas para lesão traumática) ☐
    (Código CID)                                    A = Completa    B = Sensibilidade Preservada
                                              C = Não-funcional Motora  D=Funcional Motora  E = Normal

21. OUTROS DIAGNÓSTICOS
    (Código CID)
    Mais Significativos                                 Complicações e Comorbidades
      a. _______________________         d. _______________________
      b. _______________________         e. _______________________
      c. _______________________         f. _______________________
    Diagnóstico para Transferência ou Óbito
      g. _______________________

67

# Annex 1 Inpatient assessment sheet - "MIF" (continued)

**AVALIAÇÃO DE ADMISSÃO**

22. Proveniente de  ☐

  1. Casa    2. Pensionato    3. Moradia Transitória,

  4. Casa de Repouso    5. Instalação de Cuidados Especializados

  6. UTI do próprio hospital    7. UTI de outro hospital

  8. Hospital Crônico    9. Instituição

  10. Outros    11. Óbito    12. Unidade de Cuidados Alternativos

23. Onde vivia antes de hospitalizar?  ☐

  (usar os mesmos códigos da pergunta 22)

24. Com quem vivia antes de hospitalizar?  ☐

  (Preencher apenas se respondeu "casa" na perg. 23.)

  1.Só  2. Parentes/Família  3.Amigos  4.Assistente  5.Outros

25. Ocupação antes da Hospitalização  ☐

  1. Empregado    2. Asilado    3. Estudante

  4. Dona de Casa    5. Não trabalhava

  6. Aposentado (idade)    7. Aposentado (incapacidade)

26. Carga Horária antes da hospitalização  ☐

  (Completar apenas se respondeu 1,2,3, ou 4 ao item 25)

  1.Tempo inteiro  2. Tempo parcial  3. Carga horária reduzida

**AVALIAÇÃO DE ALTA**

27. Com alta para  ☐

  1. Casa    2. Pensionato    3. Casa de Passagem

  4.Cuidados Intermédios  5. Instalação de Cuidados Especializados

  6. UTI do próprio hospital  7. UTI de outro hospital

  8. Hospital Crônico  9. Instituição de Reabilitação

  10. Outros  11. Óbito

  12. Unidade de Cuidados Alternativos de Reabilitação

28. Com alta para viver com  ☐

  ( Apenas se preenche se a resposta à perg. 27 foi "casa")

  1. Só    2. Parentes/Família    3. Amigos

  4. Assistente    5. Outros

(As perguntas 29-38 encontram-se na folha de seguimento, a seguir)

**39. MEDIDA DE INDEPENDÊNCIA FUNCIONAL (FIM)**

|  | ADMISSÃO | ALTA |
|---|---|---|
| **Cuidados com o Corpo** | | |
| A. COMER | ☐ | ☐ |
| B. APRONTAR-SE | ☐ | ☐ |
| C. BANHO | ☐ | ☐ |
| D. VESTIR PARTE SUPER. DO CORPO | ☐ | ☐ |
| E. VESTIR PARTE INFER. DO CORPO | ☐ | ☐ |
| F. TOALLET | ☐ | ☐ |
| **Controle do Esfincter** | | |
| G. CONTROLE DA BEXIGA | ☐ | ☐ |
| H. CONTROLE DO INTESTINO | ☐ | ☐ |
| **Transferência** | | |
| I. CAMA CADEIRA CADEIRA RODAS | ☐ | ☐ |
| J. SANITÁRIO | ☐ | ☐ |
| K. BANHEIRA, CHUVEIRO | ☐ | ☐ |
| **Locomoção** | | |
| L. MARCHA/CADEIRA DE RODAS (Marcha / Cad. Rod / Ambas) | ☐ | ☐ |
| M. ESCADAS | ☐ | ☐ |
| **SCORE MOTOR – SUBTOTAL** | ☐ | ☐ |
| **Comunicação** | | |
| N. COMPREENSÃO (Auditiva / Visual / Ambas) | ☐ | ☐ |
| O. EXPRESSÃO (Vocal / Não-Vocal / Ambas) | ☐ | ☐ |
| **Integração Social** | | |
| P. INTERAÇÃO SOCIAL | ☐ | ☐ |
| Q. RESOLUÇÃO DE PROBLEMAS | ☐ | ☐ |
| R. MEMÓRIA | ☐ | ☐ |
| **ESCORE COGNITIVO - SUB TOTAL** | ☐ | ☐ |
| **ESCORE TOTAL** | ☐ | ☐ |

| Níveis FIM |
|---|
| **SEM AJUDA** |
| 7 - Independência Completa |
| (Em tempo, com segurança) |
| 6 – Independência Modificada |
| (Dispositivo) |
| **COM AJUDA** |
| DEPENDÊNCIA MODIFICADA |
| 5 – Supervisão |
| 4 – Assistência Mínima |
| (O paciente realiza 75% ou +) |
| 3 – Assistência Moderada |
| (O paciente realiza 50% ou +) |
| DEPENDÊNCIA COMPLETA |
| 2 – Assistência Máxima |
| (O paciente realiza 25% ou +) |
| 1- Assistência Total |
| (O paciente realiza 0%) |

NOTA: Não deixar espaços em branco

Anote "1" se a atividade não for testada devido a riscos

# Annex 2 Term of approval of the research by the Institution

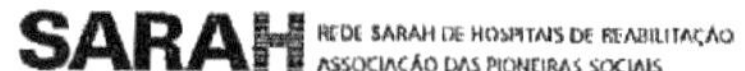

**SARAH** REDE SARAH DE HOSPITAIS DE REABILITAÇÃO
ASSOCIAÇÃO DAS PIONEIRAS SOCIAIS

**Projeto de Pesquisa/
Trabalho Científico**

Conforme O 053/2004, os trabalhos científicos devem ser
encaminhados ao Comitê de Avaliação de Trabalhos Científicos dois
meses antes da data limite estabelecida pelo evento ou periódico.

### DO PROFISSIONAL

Nome *Gerson Aguiar da Silva*

Matrícula *201519*

Cargo *Enfermeiro*    Telefone / Ramal

Admissão *03/03/93*

Área *Programa Lesado Medular*

Unidade *Fortaleza*

### DO PROJETO DE PESQUISA / TRABALHO CIENTÍFICO

O trabalho científico deverá ser anexado a este formulário, na íntegra.

As normas estabelecidas pelo periódico ou evento deverão ser seguidas. Solicita-se que uma cópia dessas normas seja anexada ao texto. Caso não haja uma norma definida, a estrutura conhecida como IMRD - Introdução, Métodos, Resultados* e Discussão*, recomendada pelo Comitê Internacional de Editores Médicos (International Comittee of Medical Journal Editors), deverá ser observada. O texto deve ser também acompanhado de resumo estruturado.

Um breve delineamento da estrutura IMRD encontra-se no anexo I. Para maior detalhamento recomenda-se a consulta à bibliografia indicada.

* Os Itens Resultados e Discussão não precisam ser preenchidos nos casos de Projetos de Pesquisa.

### DA FINALIDADE DA PESQUISA

☒ Exigência do curso de pós-graduação (anexar declaração de matrícula no curso)

Nome da Instituição de Ensino Superior *Universidade Federal do Ceará - UFC*

Curso *Mestrado em Enfermagem*

☐ Apresentação de trabalhos em eventos externos

☐ Publicação

Periódico

### DO EVENTO

Nome do Evento (por extenso)     Local

Data     Data limite de envio do trabalho (deadline)

Tipo de apresentação

☐ Poster ☐ Apresentação oral ☐ Aula ☐ Mesa Redonda ☐ Outros:

### DA CIÊNCIA DA LIDERANÇA DA ÁREA

*A temática do projeto e relevante p/ e programa do LM, pois na nossa prática a independência funcional e resultado do seu bitização.*

Data *30/12/05*     Assinatura da liderança
Linda Arair

### DA COMPROVAÇÃO

Comprometo-me a apresentar à Área de Recursos Humanos, 2(duas) cópias do trabalho para os devidos registros.

Data *30/08/05*     Assinatura do profissional

### DO PARECER DO NÚCLEO DE DIREÇÃO DA UNIDADE

☒ Favorável     ☐ Desfavorável

*De acordo.*

Data *5/1/2006*     Núcleo de Direção da Unidade

Associação das Pioneiras Sociais
Thereza Christina de Lara Alvim
Médico - CREMEC 8221

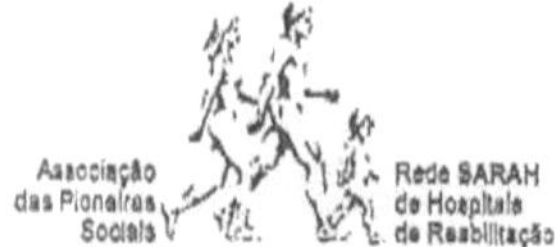

Comitê de Ética em Pesquisa da Associação das Pioneiras Sociais

## CERTIDÃO

Declaramos que o Projeto de Pesquisa, intitulado **Aplicação da medida de Independência funcional (FIM) em pessoas portadoras de paraplegia durante programa de reabilitação: resultados e fatores associados**, de **Gelson Aguiar da Silva**, cargo **Enfermeiro**, foi apreciado e considerado correto sob o ponto de vista ético pelo Comitê de Ética em Pesquisa da Rede SARAH de Hospitais de Reabilitação.

Brasília-DF, 06 de Setembro de 2006

Dr. Renato Ângelo Saraiva
Coordenador do Comitê de Ética em Pesquisa
Associação das Pioneiras Sociais

*Vianney Mesquita* (Reg. Prof. nº CE004897P)

Revisão Gramatical e Estilística de Textos
Docente da Universidade Federal do Ceará
Acad. Titular (Cad nº 37) da Acad. Cearense de Língua Portuguesa

# DECLARAÇÃO

Declaro, para constituir prova junto ao (à) PROGRAMA DE MESTRADO EM ENFERMAGEM DA UNIVERSIDADE FEDERAL DO CEARÁ,

que procedi ao trabalho de revisão estilística e gramatical do(a) DISSERTAÇÃO, intitulado(a) "INDEPENDÊNCIA FUNCIONAL DE PESSOAS PORTADORAS DE PARAPLEGIA EM PROGRAMA DE REABILITAÇÃO: RESULTADOS E FATORES ASSOCIADOS", da autoria de GERSON AGUIAR DA SILVA

orientado(a) pelo(a) PROF.ª DR.ª ZUILA M.ª F. CARVALHO, pelo que assino a presente.

Fortaleza, 19 de SETEMBRO de 2006

**Prof. João Vianney Campos de Mesquita**
Universidade Federal do Ceará e Academia Cearense da
Língua Portuguesa

# APPENDICES

**Appendix a Data collection form**

1) Age (in years):

2) Sex: ( ) male Female ( )

3) Education:

4) Date of Hospital Admission: ___/___/Date of   End Assessment: __/___/___

5) Date of Hospital Discharge: ___/___/   End Assessment Date: __/___/___

6) Hospitalisation time (in days):

7) Time since injury (until admission to the programme - in years):

8) Etiological diagnosis:

9) Classification of Spinal Cord Injury according to the ASIA Scale:

A ( ) B ( ) C ( ) D ( ) E ( )

10) Injury level (motor):

11) Complications

Pressure ulcer ( ) Spasticity ( ) OH ( ) Neuropathic pain ( ) ( ) other

# Means Plots

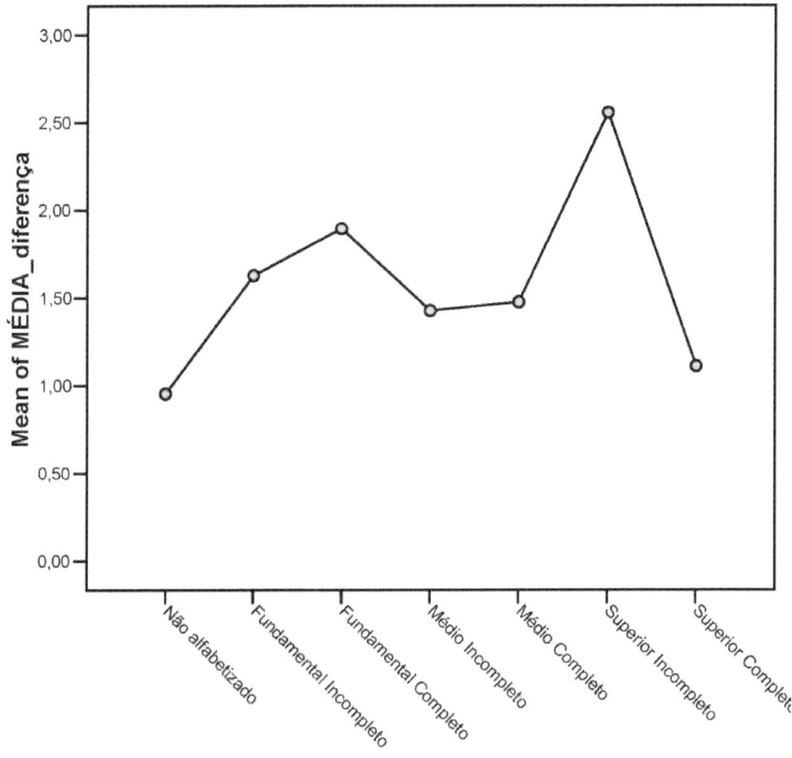


Source: National Quality Control Centre (CNCQ) - Sarah - Fortaleza - 2006

**Means Plots**

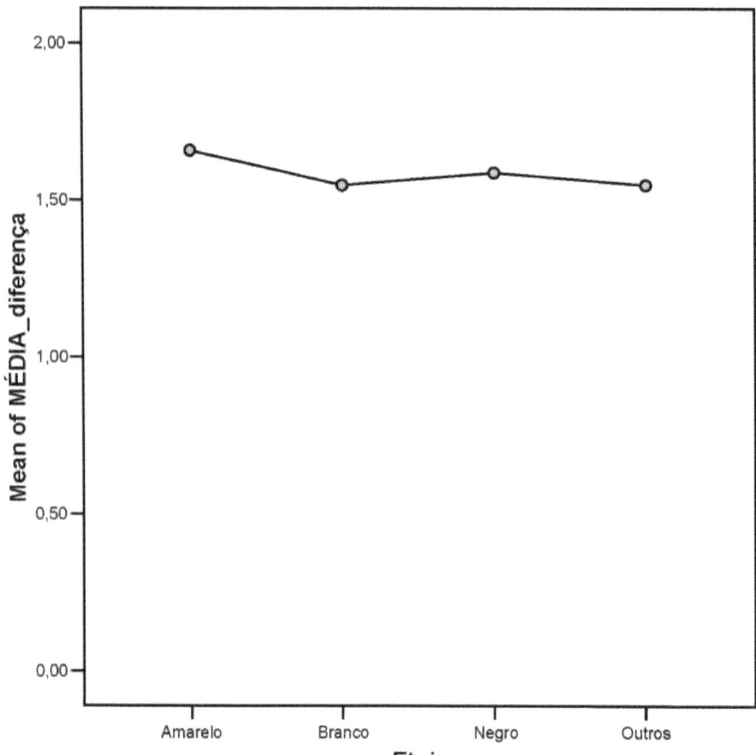


Source: National Quality Control Centre (CNCQ) - Sarah - Fortaleza - 2006

## Means Plots

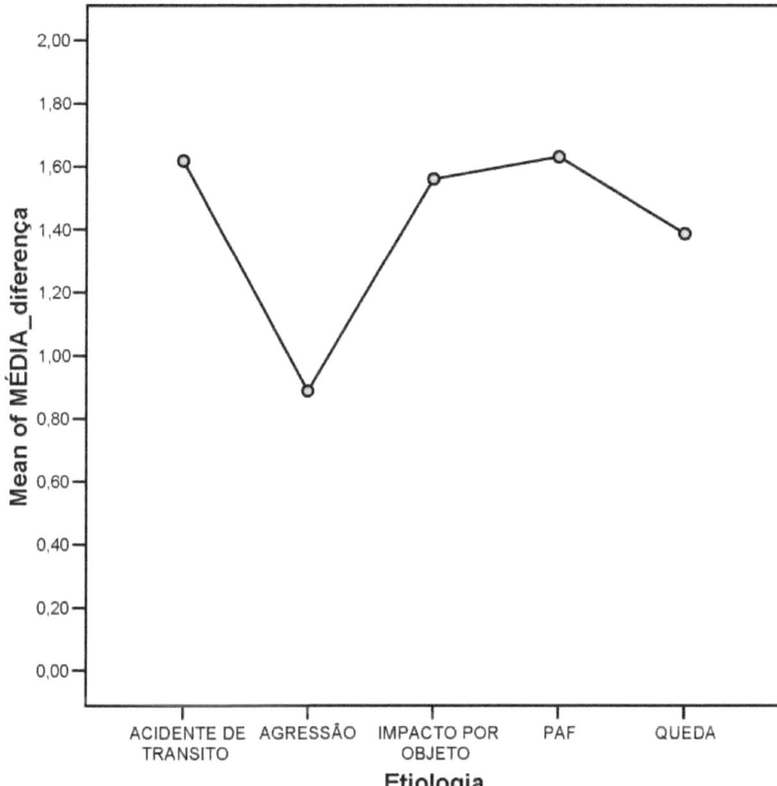



Source: National Quality Control Centre (CNCQ) - Sarah   Fortaleza - 2006

**Means Plots**

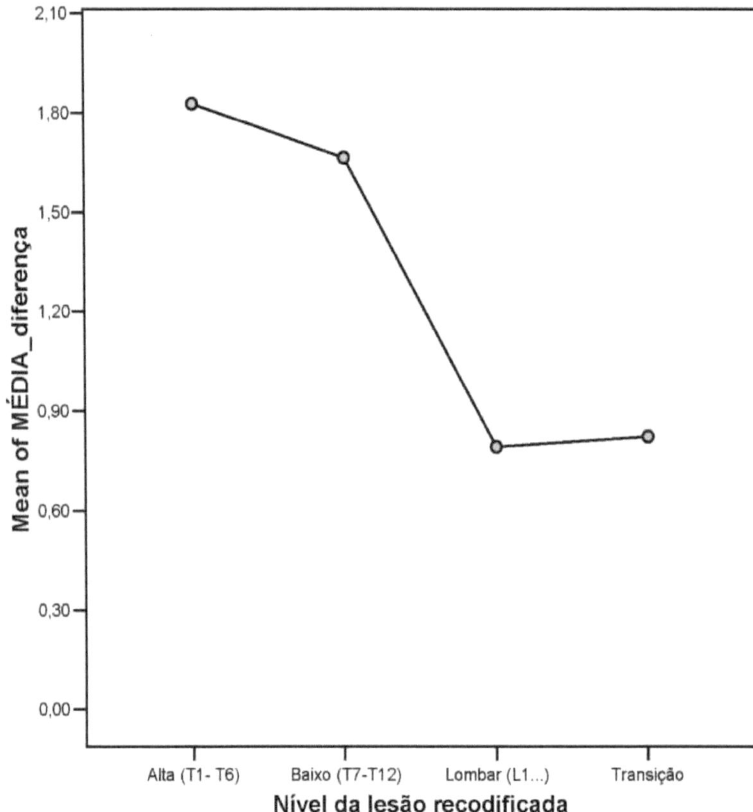


Source: National Quality Control Centre (CNCQ) - Sarah - Fortaleza - 2006

# Means Plots

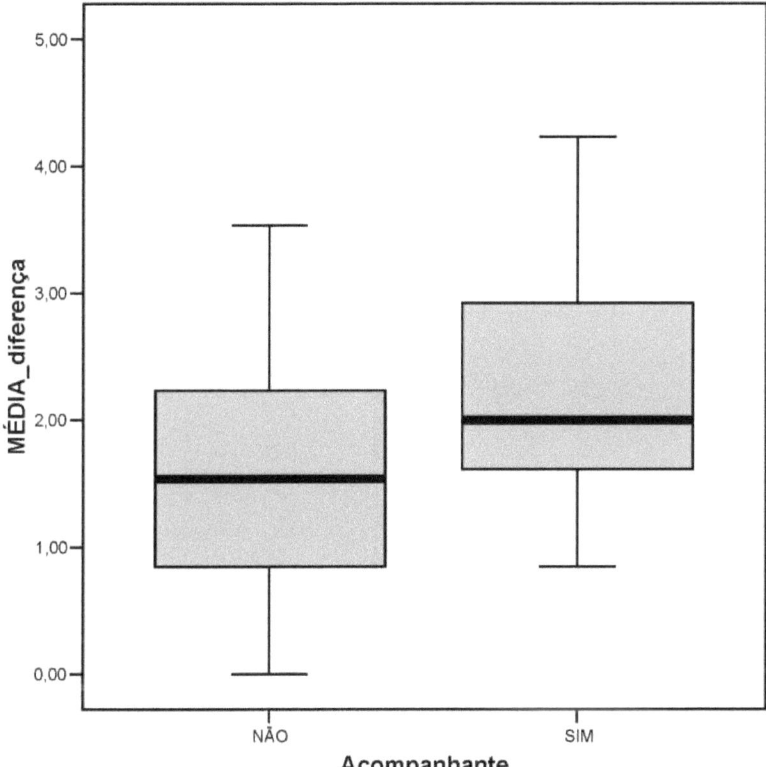


Source. National Quality Control Centre (CNCQ) - Sarah - Fortaleza - 2006

Means Plots

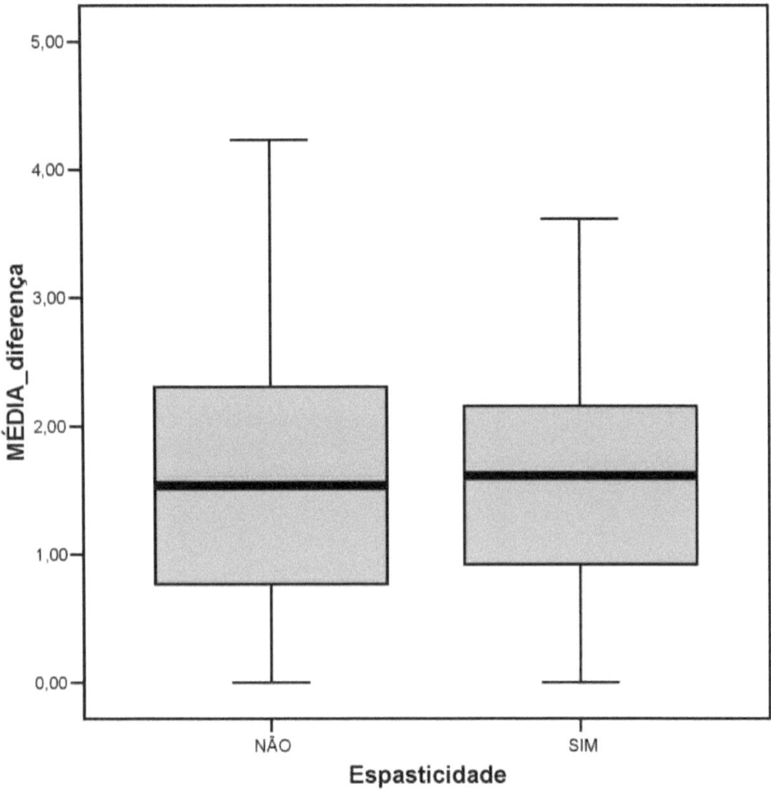


Source: National Quality Control Centre (CNCQ) - Sarah - Fortaleza - 2006

## Means Plots

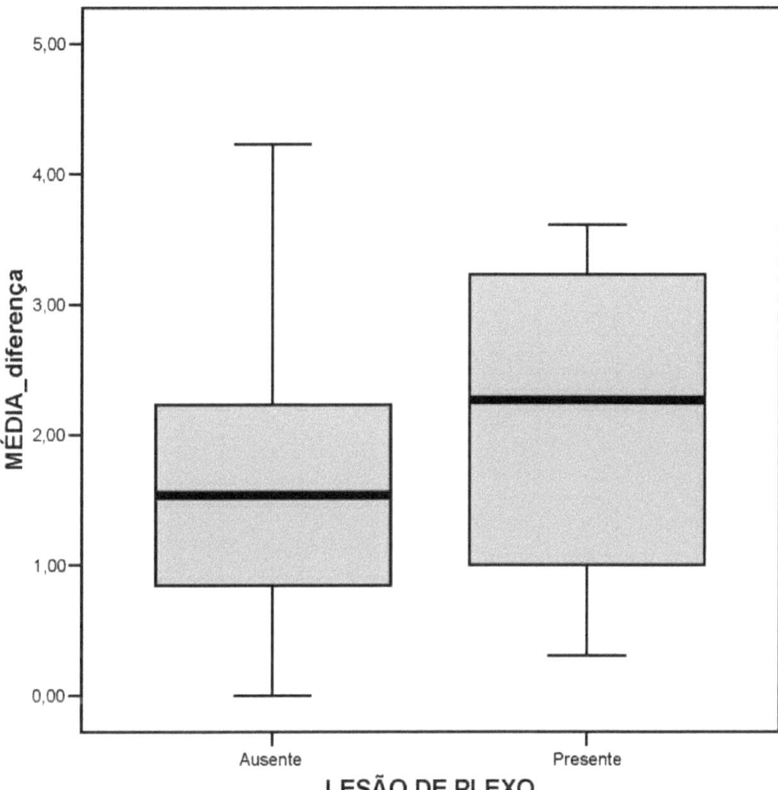



Source: National Quality Control Centre (CNCQ) - Sarah - Fortaleza - 2006

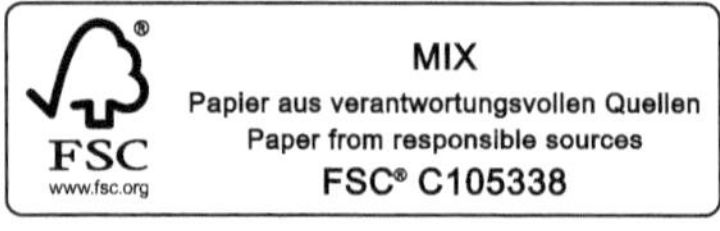


Printed by Books on Demand GmbH, Norderstedt / Germany